W9-BMP-521

— *The* —

REPETITIVE
STRAIN INJURY
RECOVERY BOOK

ALSO BY DEBORAH QUILTER

Repetitive Strain Injury: A Computer User's Guide
with coauthor Emil Pascarelli, M.D.

The REPETITIVE STRAIN INJURY RECOVERY BOOK

Deborah Quilter

FOREWORD BY
ROBERT E. MARKISON, M.D.

LAKE PARK PUBLIC LIBRARY

WALKER AND COMPANY   NEW YORK

To my students, who taught me so much.

Copyright © 1998 by Deborah Quilter

Medical disclaimer: This book is not intended to replace the advice and care of a competent physician. Rather, it is intended to help you help yourself in conjunction with a group of skilled health professionals. Your own physical condition and diagnosis may require specific modifications or precautions. Before undertaking any treatment or therapy, you should consult your physician or health-care provider. Any application of the ideas, suggestions, and procedures set forth in this book are at the reader's discretion.

All rights reserved. No part of this book may be reproduced or transmitted in any form or by any means, electronic or mechanical, including photocopying, recording, or by any information storage and retrieval system, without permission in writing from the Publisher.

The comic strip on page 26 is reprinted with special permission of King Features Syndicate. The diagram on page 28 is from HUMAN ANATOMY 2/E by Martini/Timmons © O. Reprinted by permission of Prentice-Hall, Inc., Upper Saddle River, NJ. The diagram on page 69 is reprinted with permission of Ingersoll-Rand Company. All other illustrations are by Susan Aldridge.

First published in the United States of America in 1998
by Walker Publishing Company, Inc.

Published simultaneously in Canada by Thomas Allen & Son Canada,
Limited, Markham, Ontario

Library of Congress Cataloging-in-Publication Data
Quilter, Deborah, 1950–
    The repetitive strain injury recovery book / Deborah Quilter ;
foreword by Robert E. Markison.
        p. cm.
    Includes bibliographical references and index.
    ISBN 0-8027-7514-4 (pbk.)
    1. Overuse injuries—Popular works.   2. Overuse injuries—
Prevention.   I. Title.
RD97.6.Q52 1998
617.1—dc21   97-36007
                                                        CIP

Book design by Mary Jane DiMassi

Printed in the United States of America
2   4   6   8   10   9   7   5   3   1

Contents

FOREWORD BY ROBERT E. MARKISON, M.D.   ix
PREFACE   xi
ACKNOWLEDGMENTS   xiii

1. RSI 101: AN ORIENTATION   1
   The Basics of RSI   2
   The Magnitude of the Problem   4
   The Typical Scenario   5

2. GETTING MOBILIZED: THE ACTION PLAN   11
   What You Should Do Right Away   11
   Avoid the Wrong Doctors   15
   Prioritize Your Problems   17
   Six Warnings About the Recovery Process   20

3. INJURY AND HEALING   25
   The Elements of Injury   25
   The Elements of Healing   33

4. THE EMOTIONAL ASPECTS OF RSI   41
   Common Emotional Repercussions   42
   Internet, Video, and Computer Game Addiction   47
   Interacting with Other People   47
   Steps to Emotional Healing   51
   Small Ways to Save Your Sanity   57

5. MEDICAL TREATMENTS   61
   Overview of Current Treatments   61
   The Proper RSI Examination   62
   Drug Therapy   65
   What to Consider About Surgery   68
   Types of Physical and Occupational Therapy   70
   Relapse: The Second Wave   75

6. COMPLEMENTARY AND SELF-CARE TREATMENTS   80
   Complementary Therapies   81
   Selecting What's Best for You   85
   Self-Help Techniques   86
   Cultivate Ambidexterity   90
   Relaxing Is Essential to Recovery   91
   The Relaxation Workshop: A Blueprint for Healing   91
   Four Relaxation Tips   95

7. THE HEALING POWER OF EXERCISE AND GOOD POSTURE   99
   Beginning Your Exercise Program   100
   Cautions About Exercise   105
   RSI-Friendly Exercises   107
   Activities to Avoid   108
   The Therapeutic Power of Proper Posture   108

8. PROTECTING YOUR HANDS DURING DAILY ACTIVITIES   112
   General Hand-Saving Principles   112
   The Specifics of Everyday Life   116
   Household Tips   124
   Personal Care   126
   The Telephone   127
   The Home Office   128
   On the Road with RSI   129

9. RSI AND YOUR SEX LIFE   132
   Disability Does Not End Sexuality   132
   Problems of Sexuality and Disability   133

Dating with RSI 133
Ten Ways to a Better Sex Life 136
RSI Can Bring You Closer Together 139

**10. BEYOND ERGONOMICS: SOLVING COMMON WORK-RELATED
PROBLEMS** **140**
Returning to Work After Rehabilitation 140
Protecting Your Hands at Work: Tips for the Working
Injured 142
The Proper Workstation 146
Everyone Needs a Good Chair 147
Desk Accessories 149
Keyboards and Voice Systems 151
Cautions About Risky Devices 154
The Interpersonal Aspects of Work 157
Your Job or Your Hands 158
Your Legal Alternatives 160

11. PROPER TECHNIQUE AT WORK **165**
Basic Computer Technique 166
Of Mice and Trackballs 172
Handwriting Technique 174
Voice-Activated Software 177
Advice for Musicians 179

12. CREATING YOUR NEW CAREER **183**
Deciding on a New Career 183
The Career Workshop 184
Talking About RSI on Job Interviews 188
Planning for Success 191

13. HESITATIONS ABOUT THE INFORMATION SUPERHIGHWAY **193**
The Technological Treadmill 193
The Social Consequences of Technology 195
Preventing RSI 196
The Next Generation: Children and Computer Injuries 198

EPILOGUE. DISCOVERING THE GIFTS OF RSI   203
  Gaining Perspective   203
  Rediscovering the Joys of Human Relations   205
  Discovering Who You Are and What You Want   205

  GLOSSARY   209
  REFERENCES   217
  RESOURCES   223
  FURTHER READING   231
  INDEX   233

Foreword

I am a broadly trained surgeon. I spent the first nine years of my career as a trauma surgeon and chief of hand surgery at San Francisco General Hospital treating major life- and limb-threatening injuries. Early in my career, when deciding whether to specialize in the heart or the hand, my mentor, a heart surgeon, advised, "If you want complexity, a lifelong engagement, real and true challenge, take up the hand."

I remain fascinated with my choice to this day.

The hand uses more brainpower than any other part of the body, including the heart. When the hand is unhappy, the brain is unhappy. We humans are defined by our remarkable capacity for creative hand use—consider the painting of Rembrandt and the music of Duke Ellington. One would assume that people would treat their hands as instruments worthy of great respect. One would also assume that designers would respect this precious appendage when they design tools, which is unfortunately rarely the case.

With the explosion of personal computer use in the early 1980s, I soon realized that it is more difficult to treat cumulative microtrauma than acute injury. I foresaw a steep rise in the incidence of upper-extremity strain injuries because of the combination of poor tool design and the increasingly repetitive nature of many jobs. In fact, because of this mass proliferation of poorly designed tools, repetitive strain injury has now reached epidemic proportions. Many of those injured go from doctor to doctor, often spending fruitless months until they find someone who can help them. Patients with RSI require a great deal of time, bring on mountains of paperwork, and generally do not require surgery. As a consequence, a growing number of hand surgeons and other physicians do not wish to treat this problem.

For a long time I was naive enough to think that ergonomics held the key to preventing this disease. It just isn't so. The sad fact is that many or possibly most humans are not geared to sitting at a computer all day. Too much hand use is too much hand use, even with a state-of-the-art workstation.

Nor will ergonomics alone help injured people heal. Recovery requires a much broader approach. This can include—but is not limited to—education, muscular conditioning, myofascial therapy, proper posture and breathing, a good diet, abstention from smoking and alcohol, time off work if necessary, learning to control pain without drugs, and keeping good company, by which I mean inspired and inspiring friends, a circle of friends who find magic in the ordinary and great joy in nonmaterial things; people who really can be nourishing and positive in the very best way. These methods work slowly but are frequently more effective than pills, splints, or injections, all of which tend to be overprescribed and have limited long-term effectiveness.

Despite the difficulty getting proper treatment and the enormous lifestyle changes RSI can entail, patients willing to undertake the work of recovery can do very well. Those who improvise around adversity instead of becoming mired in it can make great strides. Improvisation means being willing to make fundamental changes in what you do for a living, or how you do it. It means taking initiative instead of taking orders. This age of managed care transfers much more responsibility to the injured person.

Deborah Quilter offers sound advice about many aspects of recovery from RSI. This important and valuable book fills the gap between medical treatment and getting on with life, and is essential reading for people with RSI and especially anyone who has experienced discomfort while using a computer. She understands that we are only as good as our ability to interpret adversity and apply insight positively to our individual and collective futures. For my part, I can reassure the reader that RSI does steadily improve with appropriate care—and a healthy measure of self-tending.

—Robert E. Markison, M.D.
Associate Clinical Professor of Surgery at
the University of California–San Francisco,
and Cofounder of UCSF's Health Program
for Performing Artists

Preface

Repetitive strain injury changes your life. This condition, which attacks your body insidiously and is brought on by months and years of seemingly innocent hand movements, can result in extreme disability. Even a minor impairment of the thumb or forearm or shoulder or neck—typical sites of injury—can require major lifestyle changes. Any injury to—and healing of—the upper extremity involves the *entire* body. Because of the tendency for reinjury and the crucial importance of the hand in daily life, I believe there is no such thing as a mild case of RSI.

This knowledge comes firsthand. When I was diagnosed with RSI in 1991 I was eager to learn as much as possible in order to get better. As a longtime health writer, I knew how important it is to be an active participant in medical treatment. There was little information available on the topic, so I eventually wrote a book about RSI and began conducting workshops to share what I had learned about preventing, overcoming, and coping with RSI. Since then, new findings have come to light, more doctors have gained expertise in this area, and hundreds of RSIers have shared their experiences with me in workshops and conversations. To gain a better understanding of how the body's natural processes interact with one another, I also enrolled in a rigorous fitness certification program to study anatomy, kinesiology, physiology, and nutrition.

When beginning this book, I reviewed stacks of research studies about repetitive strain injury from many corners of the world. These reports covered topics, mainstream to esoteric, such as the rate of RSI among grocery checkers and the incidence of carpal tunnel syndrome in Alaskan fishermen.

However, none of these articles dealt with the physical, psychological, and economic realities of living with this disease. Like planes that go off the radar chart, long-term RSIers—people who have consulted doctor after doctor, lived with RSI year after year—

simply seem to drop out of sight. What becomes of them? Do they ever heal? How do they live if they can no longer work? How do they accomplish simple tasks of daily living that have become so hard to perform? How do they cope with the emotions that arise from living with a serious disability?

This book deals with the critical questions that face people who have limited use of their hands. It draws on personal experience with RSI, as well as observations from many others struggling with the difficulties RSI brought to their lives. It includes advice from many of the finest minds in this field: doctors, physical and occupational therapists, psychotherapists, and more. As might be expected, some of the most valuable insights come from the foot soldiers on the front lines, the RSIers themselves.

Many people have contributed their stories to this book. Some of them preferred not to have their names published. In those cases, they are referred to by a pseudonymous first name, with or without a last initial. Details of their stories have sometimes been changed to protect their privacy.

The focus of this book is self-care, and living with RSI over the long term. Whether you just received a diagnosis of repetitive strain injury or you have been living with RSI for several years, the very fact that you bought this book signals the beginning of healing, because you are doing the best possible thing at a critical time: arming yourself with information. The more you educate yourself about RSI—and your own unique manifestations of it—the better you will be able to take care of yourself.

Here, then, begins the odyssey. At the end, I hope you will thrive—not simply survive—with RSI.

Acknowledgments

Nonfiction authors hound librarians, haunt bookstores, and hunt experts, soaking up collective wisdom like sponges. Writers rely on others as sounding boards, soul mates, and devil's advocates. It would be too unwieldy for me to express my gratitude individually to everyone who helped me. But here is an attempt to thank a few of the many people who contributed their professional opinions, observations, expertise, and time to this book.

A quartet of doctors commented on early drafts of the manuscript:

Robert Markison, M.D., a true Renaissance man who is as comfortable wielding a saxophone or diamond saw as a scalpel, saw this epidemic coming years ago and has been way ahead of the pack ever since.

George Piligian, M.D., gave the manuscript fastidious readings.

John Cianca, M.D., lucidly illuminated many puzzling aspects of injury and healing.

Robert Rosenthal, M.D., was ever sensitive to the nuances of both language and behavior.

Others who offered suggestions for the manuscript were:

Christopher Quilter, my cousin and a gifted writer, offered much useful advice, not the least of which was telling me what the reader wanted to know.

Louis Slesin provided a gold mine of source material.

Sylvie Erb, my physical therapist, not only worked miracles with my body, she kept the faith in my recovery when my own was flagging and inspired me with her wise worldview.

Many others helped, too:

Glenn Devitt provided technical expertise, answered requests for too many favors with "No problem," and buoyed my spirits with his friendship.

Jay Goldberg, the best lawyer anyone could want, always knew the right thing to do.

Andrew Kent listened endlessly and advised me well.

Susan Nobel was especially instrumental in my decision to teach.

Emil Pascarelli, M.D., introduced me to the basic principles of repetitive strain injury, a foundation on which I continue to build.

Ellen R. Peyser, M.D., fearlessly dispensed that most potent of medicines, truth.

For help in making the book a reality:

Jonathan Dolger, my agent, helped this book become happily published; George Gibson, the publisher at Walker, had the vision to see its importance; Jacqueline Johnson, my editor at Walker, deftly guided the book through to completion with thoughtfulness, patience, and aplomb; Carol Huie brilliantly deciphered barely audible taped interviews; copy editor Vicki Haire paid careful attention to every detail; and illustrator Susan Aldridge got things just right.

For helping me verify facts: the excellent reference librarians of the New York Public Library, a national living treasure; Richard Corenthal, of Vladeck, Waldman, Elias & Engelhard, P.C., New York; Roy Goodman, Curator of Printed Materials, The American Philosophical Society; Darryl Rehr of the Early Typewriter Collectors Association; Dominick Tuminaro, of Pasternack Popish Reiff & Tuminaro, Brooklyn, New York; and all those who send me articles and papers I might not otherwise see.

I would also like to thank Merav Ben-Avi, Ann Barr, John Bloomfield, Robert Breitstein, M.D., Philip Burton, Katrina Cakuls, Mei-Nar Chou, Rehka Desai, Sue Duncan, Prudence Ferraro, Robin Mary Gillespie, Toni Golan, John Haskell, Bob Hubbard, Kathy Jalbert, Linda J. Johnson, Sefa Jorques, Susan Karp, Gary Karp, Lynda Marvin, Laura Miner, Frank Lipman, M.D., Robert Luhn, The RSI Task Force at NYCOSH, Neill Rosenfeld, Howard Ruppel, Trina Semorile, Anna Spelman, Vanessa Valdes, Tom Vasiliades, James Z. M. Wang, and Julie Weiner and the staff of the Miller Institute for Performing Artists in New York.

My friends and family were wonderfully supportive, especially

Scott Blakey, Frank Brennan, Jane Q. Kennedy, Kathryn Sullivan, Janice Tong, Joe Westmoreland, and Sheila and Dick Wheeler.

Most of all, thanks to the many RSIers who so generously shared their expertise, experiences, hopes, and dreams with me. I feel special gratitude to those RSIers whose stories appear here.

1

RSI 101: An Orientation

Repetitive strain injury starts with a whisper and ends with a scream. By the time most people realize they are injured, much damage has occurred. And, sadly, many of those afflicted will continue to get worse until they can find a physician with enough understanding about the complexities of the upper extremity to diagnose and prescribe helpful treatment.

Because people have no idea what the warning signs of injury are, they do not have a chance to protect themselves. Warning signs can be subtle—a vague awareness of your hands or unaccustomed clumsiness—or obvious—shooting pains or loss of the ability to snap your fingers.

RSI can affect the neck, shoulders, upper back, upper arm, elbows, forearms, wrists, or fingers, so warning signs of injury can occur in any of these areas. Here are the most common warning signs:

- Weakness in the hands or forearms
- Fatigue
- Lack of endurance
- Tingling, numbness, or loss of sensation
- A feeling of heaviness in your arms
- Frequent clumsiness
- Difficulty opening and closing hands
- Stiffness in hands
- Difficulty using hands (i.e., trouble turning pages of books or magazines, twisting doorknobs or faucets, holding a coffee mug, buttoning clothing, or putting on jewelry)

- Reluctance to shake hands
- Difficulty carrying things or holding bus or subway poles
- Hands falling asleep
- Waking up with wrist pain or numb hands, especially during early-morning hours
- Lack of control or coordination
- Cold hands
- Frequent self-massage
- Soreness or mild to excruciating pain, which can be dull, achy, electrical, stabbing
- Tremors
- Avoidance of sports or other activities that were once enjoyable

Being diagnosed with RSI has many of the nightmarish qualities of the first week of college. You come to a new campus, surrounded by strangers, search for your classroom hoping you don't walk in late. You meet your professors, look at the reading list, and think you'll never learn all they expect you to know. With RSI, you enter a strange new world of puzzling symptoms, where doctors use scary-sounding medical terms and you sometimes receive conflicting advice. No wonder you feel shell-shocked.

Everybody should receive a basic orientation to this disease. Your physician may not have the time to tell you all you need to know, but there is a lot you can learn on your own. Here is a brief summary about RSI. Check the glossary in this book for explanations of the medical terms used.

The Basics of RSI

"The underlying premise for the term 'CTD' [cumulative trauma disorders, another term for RSI] is that tissues that would normally be able to withstand the stresses to which they are exposed during a work activity eventually become diseased because they experience repeated *exposure with insufficient time in between exposures to heal properly*. Over the long term, the relatively innocuous work task, and other similar tasks, become difficult or impossible to perform," writes Ann Barr, assistant professor of the Department of Physical Therapy at Temple University in Philadelphia.

Five Things to Know Right Away

• **Repetitive strain injury is frequently chronic.** If it is, you cannot go back to the way things were before your injury. To heal, you will need to modify how you use your hands in every aspect of your life.

• **Healing takes time.** Progress is often slow with RSI, but you can make a remarkable recovery. Rushing your recovery may result in relapses.

• **Recovery requires work.** There is no magic pill for RSI, but if you are willing to make the effort, you can reduce pain and regain some use of your hands.

• **Every treatment does not work for every body.** You may try an array of treatments with varying results. You will be the final authority about what helps, because you know your body best.

• **You can change the outcome.** You can enlist the aid of many doctors and other health professionals, but ultimately much of the progress you make will depend on how well you take care of your body. By making positive choices about how you use your hands, you can influence the healing process.

"Repetitive strain injury" is a collective term that refers to many separate ailments affecting the nerve, muscles, tendons, and vasculature of the hand, wrist, arm, neck, and shoulder. Since the hand and arm are connected to the neck and upper back, the strain can spread into different areas; thus most people have several diagnoses instead of just one. Other terms for RSI include "occupational overuse injuries" and "cumulative trauma disorders." While other areas of the body—such as the back, knees, and feet—can suffer overuse injuries, here the term "RSI" is reserved for injuries to the upper extremity.

Symptoms of RSI include numbness, tingling, lack of endurance, tremor, clumsiness, lack of sensation, a feeling of heaviness, and pain. People can experience pain at rest or during activity—anywhere along the hand, arm, shoulder, or neck. Pain can be burning, achy, sore, or jolting, like an electrical shock; it can range from mild to excruciating. People should seek medical evaluation immediately if they experience any warning signs of RSI—even if they are mild, or symptoms come and go, as they do in Stage 1 injury. If they wait until they have more severe symptoms, it may be too late to prevent chronic problems.

Any repetitive use of the hand can be problematic; therefore RSI occurs in professions as diverse as dentistry and data processing, music making and meatpacking, calligraphy and carpentry.

Injury happens over months and years, and once it has occurred even minor use of the hand can be troublesome. Recovery is most often a slow and arduous process.

Nerve injuries include: carpal tunnel syndrome, radial tunnel syndrome, cubital tunnel syndrome, Guyon's canal syndrome, sulcus ulnaris tunnel syndrome, and others.

Muscle and tendon injuries include: myofascial pain, tenosynovitis, epicondylitis, De Quervain's disease, trigger finger, bicipital tendinitis, rotator cuff tendinitis, flexor carpi radialis tendinitis, extensor tendinitis, flexor tendinitis, and others.

Other common injuries include cervical radiculopathy, thoracic outlet syndrome, Raynaud's disease, and focal dystonia.

Conditions such as degenerative joint disease (osteoarthritis), fibromyalgia, and Dupuytren's contracture can complicate RSI.

The Magnitude of the Problem

Repetitive strain injury has swept the nation. According to the Bureau of Labor Statistics, it accounts for 62 percent of all work-related ailments—more than any other occupational disease. Some of these people become permanently disabled, and it is unlikely they will ever work again. Relatively young, formerly productive workers wind up on Workers' Compensation rolls, public assistance programs, and employers' disability insurance programs.

According to the Bureau of Labor Statistics, there were 23,000 cases of RSI in 1981. The number has grown steadily. There were 332,000 new cases in 1994 alone. In 1995, the number dipped slightly to 308,000. To get an idea of the relative size of the problem, consider the estimates from 1995 for the leading kinds of cancer in the United States: lung cancer (169,900 cases per year), breast cancer (183,400), colorectal cancer (138,200), and prostate cancer (244,000). According to the Occupational Safety and Health Administration (OSHA), 2.7 million Workers' Compensation claims for RSI were paid in 1993, two-thirds of which were for back injuries, and the remainder—910,000 claims—were for upper-extremity injuries.

As staggering as it is, this number may be low. The National Institute for Occupational Safety and Health (NIOSH) discovered that the BLS had underestimated the number of cases. A University of California study found that only 44 percent of work-related injuries were reported and suggested that the incidence rate may be 130 percent higher than those counted.

According to OSHA, the estimated cost to business in 1993 alone was $120 billion.

Who gets injured? People who use their hands repetitively. Computer users, carpenters, dentists, plumbers, letter sorters, data entry clerks, graphic designers, checkout clerks, jewelers, and butchers can all develop RSI. According to a study of sign language interpreters, in 1990, 60 percent of forty-two full-time interpreters at the National Technical Institute for the Deaf were diagnosed with a work-related tendinitis or nerve entrapment disorder such as carpal tunnel syndrome. (This finding was reported by Michael Feuerstein and Terence E. Fitzgerald in the *Journal of Occupational Medicine.*)

The Typical Scenario

Repetitive strain injury is primarily a disease of ignorance. We take our hands for granted—indeed, people are often very surprised to discover that hands can become crippled from overuse. They as-

The Stages of Injury

STAGE 1
- Pain and fatigue near the end of the workday
- Symptoms resolve overnight and on days off
- No reduction in work performance
- Condition lasts weeks or months
- Injury reversible

STAGE 2
- Recurrent pain and fatigue earlier in the workday
- Night symptoms cause sleep disturbance
- Reduced work capacity
- Physical signs such as swelling or positive reactions to provocative tests such as Tinel's Sign or a nerve conduction study. At this stage, the physical signs may be more discernible to a knowledgeable doctor than to the patient.
- Condition persists for months
- Possibly reversible

sume that office work is "safe," that it's impossible to become disabled from sitting at a desk using a computer or making small movements with your hands. But let's look at how easily that could happen in a composite scenario based on many real-life examples.

Day in, day out, you arrive at your office, log on to your computer, and spend most of the following eight hours sitting, making tiny hand movements or holding rigidly still while you stare at the screen. Hour after hour, your neck bends down while you read or write, the weight of your head pulling your shoulders forward, straining the muscles of the upper back. Tiny microtears mar the soft tissue. Scar tissue, which is less elastic than muscle tissue, develops. The muscle tightens, a reaction to the damage, and now works less efficiently because range of motion is diminished.

STAGE 3
- Pain and fatigue even during rest and nonrepetitive movement
- Night pain causes sleep disturbance
- Reduced work capacity
- Condition lasts months to years
- Reversibility unlikely

RED FLAGS
- Numbness, tingling, or burning
- Weakness or clumsiness
- Night symptoms
- Persistent symptoms
- Pain-related behaviors, such as frequent self-massage; protective postures; aversion to touch; wincing and moaning; guarding the affected area

The muscles that work the arm and hand become weaker and weaker, but this weakness is usually not noticed until after pain develops, which may take many months or years.

WORKING IN PAIN

Many people live in a great deal of job-related pain. You get neck aches, and pain in your shoulders, forearms, thumbs, and wrists, but you may not associate these signs with your work. Instead, you attribute them to the fact that you're getting older, or to another activity, such as painting the apartment or playing tennis. But the real culprit is how you use your hands every day, making tiny repetitive movements or holding still for long periods of time, or lack of exercise. Frequent computer use is an athletic activity for which many people are physically unprepared.

While the microtrauma can take years to develop into full-blown injury, people usually associate it with one or two dramatic events. One man who worked as a programmer said his hands gave out after working one hundred hours a week on a rush project. This may have been what triggered his current crisis, but his injury was long in the making. RSI does not happen overnight; it sneaks up on you insidiously.

DENYING THE INJURY

Instead of taking the body's warnings seriously, many people deny they are injured, especially when symptoms come and go. Some people even disregard excruciating pain while performing important daily tasks such as dressing, brushing their teeth, or driving. This denial can last an extraordinarily long time. People who find it agonizing to sign a check insist on staying at their jobs—working in intense pain—rather than taking time off to let their body heal.

Sometimes people seek help only when their hands give out on them and they can no longer force their hands to work despite the pain. By that time, their injury has reached stage 3 (see box on pages 6–7).

ATTEMPTS AT SELF-MEDICATION

You may try to treat yourself for chronic pain instead of seeking professional help. You go on vacation and think your hands have recovered because they are pain-free. But your symptoms recur within five minutes of returning to work. You buy pillows or wrist pads or an "ergonomic" chair. You use splints, take over-the-counter drugs, or visit chiropractors or acupuncturists to quell the pain. Some people double or triple pain medication just to get through the day; yet this practice can be harmful.

Pain is a signal that you need to stop the offensive activity. Masking pain—while continuing to abuse your hands—can make your injury more severe.

HIDING THE INJURY

When people have a skating accident, or catch the flu that's going around, they usually commiserate with their colleagues at work.

However, people with RSI frequently keep their condition a secret. There are a number of reasons for this.

Staff-level office workers may not dare ask for workstation accommodations because they fear losing their jobs. They may not ask for a lighter workload or take more frequent breaks because they are afraid that if their productivity falls off, they may be terminated. Losing one's job is a legitimate fear, but continuing to work at the same pace may lead to permanent, severe disability later on.

Many executive-level RSIers also hide their injury. Because of corporate downsizing, executives who used to dictate to secretaries are now expected to do their own computer work. In order to hide their injury from management, many executives seek private medical treatment rather than enter the Workers' Compensation system, unaware that if their injury is work-related, their health insurer can contest the claim.

If you are self-employed, you also have to contend with intense pressures. You cannot fall back on the Workers' Compensation system to pay for your medical care. And unless you have disability insurance, you lose your income while you recuperate.

FACING POSSIBLE DISABILITY

If people do not address their injuries early, sooner or later they can make a terrifying discovery. Before, if you stopped working, your hands stopped hurting. Now, despite the fact that you have stopped working, the injury may continue. *Any* use of your hand may be troublesome. The simple act of reaching for something may hurt; turning a doorknob may be excruciating.

In addition to physical pain, you experience skyrocketing anxiety when you can't use your hands. This anxiety is perfectly understandable: Your life and emotions spiral out of control if you are no longer able to earn a living, or do even the most basic life tasks for yourself without difficulty.

Many RSIers must also deal with pressures of the Workers' Compensation system. While it is fortunate that some people have this insurance to cover their medical costs, claimants are often treated like criminals instead of injured patients who need assistance and skilled treatment.

PICKING UP THE PIECES

Chronic RSI does not necessarily lead to unemployment, financial ruin, and emotional turmoil. You can stop the ravages of RSI and slowly begin to put your life in order again. This is best done in a patient, methodical way. First, you need an accurate diagnosis and proper medical treatment. Then you need to educate yourself about exercise, proper posture, and self-care, with emphasis on the importance of awareness and attitude. When you are ready to return to work, you need instruction about pacing, proper workstation setup, and tools. *All* of these areas must be addressed for healing and recovery to occur.

2

GETTING MOBILIZED:
THE ACTION PLAN

When people realize how serious RSI is, they usually want to solve all their problems immediately, yet they don't know where to go or what to believe. For most, finding proper treatment is a haphazard mix of trial and error. There is no surefire way to avoid mistakes, but taking certain actions—and being aware of some pitfalls—can help.

What You Should Do Right Away

Of all the soft tissue injuries, the hand presents the greatest disability when impaired.
—RENE CAILLIET, M.D.

The first thing to do is face up to the problem, the sooner the better. Denying and/or hiding an injury is all too common. Some people try to fix matters themselves—by getting massages, self-splinting, or buying ergonomic aids—which only serves to worsen the situation by prolonging the early stage of RSI and, thus, risking chronic injury.

After people admit that they are having problems with their hands, they want to do something right away to stop their symptoms. One woman called me in a lather, saying she wanted to know what she could do right *now*. "I'm going to go to the drugstore and buy splints," she announced, unaware that self-splinting could significantly worsen this condition.

Other people find out that their muscles are weak and begin doing hand exercises such as squeezing rubber balls or performing wrist curls with weights. That's another bad idea, because this further stresses inflamed tissues.

Instead of rushing out and trying to instantly solve your problem—which was probably many years in the making—the best thing to do is calmly take stock of your situation and devise a plan. You can also help yourself by discontinuing any activity that aggravates your symptoms until you get sound medical advice. This may mean taking time off work until you see a doctor.

SEEK COMPETENT MEDICAL CARE

Don't put off seeing your doctor when you have symptoms because you assume there's nothing your doctor can do.

This is not true—provided you see a competent physician who understands how to diagnose your injury. Proper physical therapy can reduce pain, improve range of motion, and help you increase strength and endurance. The longer you put off getting treatment for a nagging injury, the greater the risk of far more serious problems down the line.

Another man presumed all cases of RSI would be treated the same way and shrugged off a suggestion that he seek a medical evaluation instead of simply having massages for his symptoms. "Why should I see a doctor? The treatment will be the same one way or the other." There may be some similarities in approach, but with an astute physician, treatment will differ depending on the diagnosis. Certain exercises can be good for one kind of RSI and contraindicated in others. You could also have an underlying medical problem that needs treatment.

SELECT A *GOOD* DOCTOR

Repetitive strain injury is a very complex disease. You need a doctor who is not only expert in soft tissue injuries, which are poorly understood even among medical professionals, but who is also willing to listen, guide, and support you through difficult emotional, financial, and physical battles.

Unfortunately, many doctors are not trained to diagnose and treat RSI, and patients' injuries can worsen until they find a competent physician. A father of three children was summarily told, "Oh, you have mild carpal tunnel syndrome. We don't have to do surgery yet." His doctor offered no guidance on limiting or reversing his injury. One woman said her physician could not find anything wrong, so he referred her to a psychiatrist. She later received a clear-cut diagnosis of tendinitis from another doctor. There is certainly a place for psychological treatment with RSI—such as dealing with the emotional fallout of losing full use of your hands, your job, and your ability to care for yourself—but not as a substitute for competent physical treatment.

Neill Rosenfeld, a former newspaper reporter, had to educate his primary-care physician about RSI and convince him there was a problem. "It took a good deal of nagging until he finally sent me to an orthopedist," Neill said. "The orthopedist told me there was no such thing as RSI, it was all in my head. I said, 'Excuse me, it's not all in my head, it's in my hands!' I sent a complaint to my HMO saying 'educate your doctors.' As a result, I got referred to a rheumatologist, who had heard of RSI." Unfortunately, according to Neill, the rheumatologist's method of treatment left something to be desired: He wrote Neill an open-ended prescription for an anti-inflammatory drug. Neill happened to mention this to a pharmacist he knew, who advised that the drug should not be taken for more than three months at a time. "This could wreck your stomach," the pharmacist warned.

Some doctors send people for X rays or MRIs, but soft tissue injuries will not necessarily show up on these tests. "A negative MRI does not mean there is not soft tissue damage," said Dr. George Piligian, an occupational health physician at Mount Sinai's Irving J. Selikoff Center for Occupational and Environmental Medicine in New York City. "The validity of the test can depend on technique, interpretation, and the inherent limitation of MRI testing itself." To compound the problem of getting adequate treatment, many doctors refuse to take Workers' Compensation patients. This is understandable, given the enormous volume of paperwork and long wait to be paid, but it makes it harder for patients to find good care.

Because RSI affects nerves, muscles, and soft tissue, you may need a specialist to get a precise diagnosis. Unfortunately, since this is an emerging field, you cannot always rely on specialists in certain branches of medicine to have current knowledge about RSI. However, occupational physicians, physiatrists (physical medicine specialists), and sports medicine doctors will be more likely to have experience with it than will other specialists.

Dr. Piligian advises that you look for a physician with these qualifications: experience and interest in RSI, affiliation with a teaching hospital, certification by the American Board of Medical Specialties,

---

Checklist for Doctor's Visit

Before you see your doctor, prepare yourself. Call and find out whether the physician accepts Workers' Compensation insurance; otherwise your visit may not be covered by it. Bring a list of your symptoms, test results, diagnoses by other doctors, and treatments and medications they have prescribed. Note how effective—or ineffective—those treatments and medications have been. Write down questions so you will not forget to ask them. For example:

- Are there any restrictions at work? Should I request light duty? (If so, get a note for your employer.)
- Do I need any modifications to my workstation (special chair, headset, keyboard tray)? Bring a picture or videotape of your workstation to your doctor.
- Should I take time off from work?
- Should I think of a new career?

If you are insecure about dealing with doctors, ask a friend to accompany you to your office visit.

and—this is very important—success in treating other RSIers. Ask around. If several people rave about a doctor, chances are, he or she is good.

What do you look for in a doctor? You want a physician who will treat your fears as well as your physical ailments, who will teach as well as treat you, sympathize when you suffer, and rejoice with you when you improve.

Competence. More than a few RSIers have said that until they showed up, their doctor had never heard of RSI.

Thoroughness. Your doctor should lay her hands on you and test the muscles that work the fingers and arms. She should observe postural imbalances and ask about past accidents and injuries, your general health, diet, working conditions, and state of mind.

Openness to your ideas. Is your doctor willing to listen to your ideas about treatment? In the early stages of her injury, April S. realized massage was very helpful to her and asked her doctor to prescribe it. He refused, questioning her need for massage. Another physician might have been delighted to help April get treatment that benefited her.

This open-mindedness is particularly important if you are using alternative healing approaches for your RSI. Your doctor should know about these treatments so he can advise you about potential complications. If you do not trust your doctor, you may not volunteer this information.

Concern and compassion. There is no miracle drug for RSI; however, by merely listening—and understanding your situation—a doctor can lift a huge load from your heavy heart. Your relatives or friends may not comprehend what you are going through, but your doctor knows—and can verify that this isn't all in your head.

Sometimes a doctor will make you feel better almost instantly just by his concerned, attentive demeanor. This is generally a pretty accurate indication that you and your doctor will get along well. In the best doctor-patient relationships, patients become partners with their doctors, instead of being helplessly dependent on them.

Avoid the Wrong Doctors

There are many fine physicians in practice all over the country. However, some RSIers have had trouble getting proper treatment.

It helps to be aware of problem doctors, so you can seek other opinions if necessary.

Watch out for doctors who predict the worst. As Dr. Andrew Weil pointed out in *Spontaneous Healing,* a doctor's attitude can have a huge impact on patients. Dr. Weil maintains that doctors who make negative statements such as "There is nothing you can do" or "You just have to live with this" are "hexing" their patients.

Dr. Robert Markison, a hand surgeon in San Francisco, concurred: "The hopeless doctor will never give hope to the patient."

Another type of problem doctor is the sadist. Lynette C., a writer, visited a hand specialist who said, after a cursory examination, "You'll never write again. You'll live in constant pain for the rest of your life, so you better get used to it."

"He didn't say anything about follow-up appointments," Lynette said. "You don't tell someone they'll never write again and then see them to the door. It was cruel. I'm sure he's seen people with their hands cut off, so to him RSI may seem like a luxury.

"I told a psychotherapist about it, and she said he was a clear-cut sadist. She said doctors who are guided by sadism instead of medical wisdom often give incorrect diagnoses."

Indeed, the doctor erred in his assessment of Lynette, who is doing very well in recovery. She progressed from a time when slicing a banana caused excruciating pain to having only occasional achiness when her wrists are tired. Fortunately, she did not allow herself to be hexed by her doctor's negative attitude.

The third type of problem doctor is the sexist or paternalist. As *New York Times* columnist Jane Brody noted, "When a disease is uncommon, its symptoms diffuse and its usual victims female, the correct diagnosis is too often overlooked by one doctor after another and patients are labeled nuisances or referred to psychiatrists."

One woman described her doctor as cold, and unresponsive to her requests. "He hardly talked to me, hardly looked at my hand." Finally, he looked at her forearm and said, "What are you going to do about that hair there?" The woman was so stunned she couldn't say a word.

Prioritize Your Problems

It is not uncommon for newly diagnosed RSIers to misorder their priorities as they realize how serious their problem is. One woman complained that her coworkers did not believe she was injured and she had a hard time delegating hand-intensive work. She refused to take a leave of absence from her job, so she continued the activities that caused her great pain.

A better action plan would have been to take time off work to rest her injury and evaluate her situation, focusing on one problem at a time. Then she could plan a safe return to work or look at different career options.

CONSIDER TAKING TIME OFF FROM WORK

The first step toward recovery is becoming pain-free, which usually involves rest. If your employer can provide a job that does not aggravate your injury, it is probably better for your frame of mind to keep working. If you cannot resist the urge to push yourself through pain and soreness, however, it would be better if you took time off.

Forcing yourself to work through pain can have disastrous consequences. During the acute stage of injury, one woman who was planning to take some time off decided to work *more* hours per week to make up for the income she would lose while she recuperated, a big mistake. Working longer and harder than ever when you are in pain can mean the difference between a reversible injury and a chronic one.

TAKE *REGULAR* BREAKS

In the beginning, RSIers typically think, "Oh, I'll do just ten more minutes," instead of taking their scheduled breaks. They lift something they know is too heavy or perform other hand-intensive tasks, only to find out, too late, that it triggers a relapse.

Pain is a warning signal from the body. If you feel pain or soreness, attend to it at once. By stopping *before* you feel pain, you can keep yourself pain-free and assist in the healing process. Don't wait until you are in pain.

Kate's Story

Kate M. is a computer troubleshooter and technology manager for a large bank. She had an unsettling experience with an insurance company doctor.

When I first walked in, he seemed to have some sort of attitude. I told him I was in pain, and he waved his hand, like *So what?*

He didn't want to hear about my neck. He said if I had the tendon in my wrist operated on that would take care of the pain in my neck. Then he examined me. He told me to put my head up and down. I told him I couldn't, so he pushed my head for me. He did the same thing with my wrist and arms. I kept saying I was in pain, and he kept waving it away. He wrote down the angles of where he was pushing me on my chart, not what I was able to do on my own.

He said, "What would you like?" I said I wanted to

With RSI, partial measures do not work. You counteract the benefits of physical therapy if you continue working at a breakneck pace while in pain. Take frequent breaks, or stop work entirely if you are sore.

DON'T LET OTHER PEOPLE FORCE YOUR HAND

It is bad enough that RSIers tend to push themselves too hard, but they can also get into trouble when they allow other people to pressure them. People who do not understand the fragility of your hands might unwittingly ask you to do things that are dangerous.

You know your limitations. Don't let anyone push you. If other people are impatient for you to heal, do not feel pressured. Also get healthy. I wanted to get back to where I was before this happened—to go grocery shopping, clean up my apartment, and blow-dry my hair. He said, "You may never be able to do the things you did before, but that's life."

Then he told a story about this kid he knew who was going to school, graduated with honors, and began looking for a job. [The kid] interviewed with a company and got a good position. He made a big point that the kid got everything because he knew someone who could help him get ahead, "Just like you."

I really got the feeling that it was a case of, You do something for me and I'll help you out. I was very, very uncomfortable. It sounded like the doctor was expecting something. It's not that he did anything overt, but to this day, I know he was after something.

People go to doctors, trusting them for help. You go there expecting them to take care of you. You don't expect any advances or anything unethical or unprofessional.

resist the temptation to compare yourself with other RSIers who might be capable of doing more than you can. Each case of RSI is unique.

AVOID COMPLACENCY

In early recovery, people generally ignore pleas to pace themselves. You think because you are now out of pain, you can use your hands the way you once did. So you plunge into work full tilt and come down with a roaring relapse.

Little by little, though, your hands teach you. You learn not to push. You stop before becoming symptomatic.

You also stop being dazzled by technology. A man who once

loved computer innovations remarked sadly, "This isn't fun anymore." No activity that causes pain and disability will be enjoyable.

When your hands get better, do not forget everything you have learned. Some people must repeat the cycle of injury and reinjury many times before they learn to be vigilant.

BEWARE OF UNRELIABLE INFORMATION

After they are injured, most people read everything they can get their hands on about RSI. While educating yourself about your medical condition is one of the best things you can do, be careful about the source of that information. At present, even many physicians do not understand how to diagnose and treat this disease, and not all "ergonomists" have appropriate experience and credentials.

Perhaps because of their mistrust of the medical establishment, many people seek advice from on-line support groups. Other members sometimes offer well-intentioned but erroneous advice, which could be counterproductive, if not dangerous. Remember, the people in such listserves are not doctors. Most physicians prefer to see a patient in person so they can perform a thorough evaluation and get a complete medical history. A single question—out of context of the medical history of the person posing it—posted on a bulletin board cannot be responsibly answered. Some vendors use the groups to advertise products and services, which may or may not be of value.

This is not to say that the RSI usenet groups are not valuable. They allow people to share resources and information as well as offer emotional support to one another.

Six Warnings About the Recovery Process

RSI is not like garden-variety aches and pains that come and go, and many people are very surprised to discover that their hands do not recovery quickly. This injury may have developed over many months or years; it will take time and patience to begin healing.

While there are very good treatments that will reduce pain and help you regain some strength, they will not necessarily restore your limbs to the state they were in prior to your injury.

Even after becoming free of pain, some people are disappointed that years later they still have not recovered full function of their hands. They may be able to use their hands for certain activities, but they find they have less endurance than they had before their injury. Many RSIers must protect their hands against reinjury for the rest of their lives.

NO ONE HAS ALL THE ANSWERS

New knowledge about repetitive strain injury is emerging every day. No single physician could possibly keep up with the entire field, so doctors should not be faulted for not knowing all there is to know. It takes a lot of time to learn how to diagnose and treat RSI, noted Dr. Piligian. "Doctors keep learning, and the best anyone can say is, 'This is how much we know today.'"

This very statement offers us all great hope: As the collective wisdom grows, we will all benefit.

PAIN-FREE DOES NOT MEAN INJURY-FREE

Repetitive strain injury "hides." Just because you don't have active symptoms does not mean you are cured forever. You will discover that you will have good days and bad days: Sometimes—often for no apparent reason—your hands will feel better than at other times. Learn to respect your limits so you do not turn a minor flare-up into a major setback.

NEW TECHNOLOGIES WILL NOT NECESSARILY SOLVE RSI

During lectures about RSI, audience members generally show great interest in "ergonomic" keyboards, chairs, and voice dictation programs, overlooking the most important component of all: what kind of shape their body is in.

Because of a general lack of understanding about the human body, people assume another kind of input device will make their problems disappear. Consider, for a moment, some common risk factors for RSI: speed, because the muscles fatigue from going too fast for prolonged periods; stress, which can stem from job-related or personal problems; repetition, because constantly using the same small muscles again and again fatigues them; faulty technique, such as wrist-resting, a common habit with computer users; sedentary behavior, which is basically a lack of regular exercise; poor physical conditioning, again from lack of exercise; and poor posture. Not a single device on the market solves these problems.

New technology cannot save you if it simply shifts the burden of work to another body part. It also means spending more money on new equipment that may in turn require different workstation configurations and, most frustrating of all, spending weeks or months becoming proficient with a new program.

BEWARE OF RSI "CURES"

No one is more interested in cures for RSI than people who have it. But so far, people who claim to have cures are sadly misinformed or just out to make a quick buck. Repetitive strain injury cannot be treated with one simple (or simpleminded) solution.

A woman once told me that she had been having trouble with carpal tunnel syndrome, then whipped out of her purse a blue wristband that contained a magnet. "This saved me," she said. If wearing a magnet made her feel better, great—so long as her doctor was aware of what she was doing, and she was getting appropriate medical treatment. But how will a magnet protect her from improper technique, poor posture, or overwork?

Many people make similar claims about vitamin supplements, herbal preparations, or new keyboards. What they do not realize is that in the early stages of injury, RSI is episodic. You have bouts of pain that eventually subside. Someone may attribute a remission of symptoms to a new vitamin or gadget. If you continue the offending behavior, the pain and symptoms will eventually stop going away, and you will be in worse shape than you would be in had you sought competent medical advice in the first place.

The notion of a cure for RSI always makes me somewhat uncomfortable, because it doesn't take into account the complexity of this disease. To some people, the word "cure" means they can start abusing their hands again.

I do not mean to imply that RSI is hopeless. People can do very well in recovery when they follow the proper protocols. And some-

Situations That Require Caution

When you injure your hands, you may need to use caution in situations you never thought twice about before your injury.

- **Driving.** Driving can aggravate RSI, and some people stop this activity if their hands fall asleep, if they have trouble keeping a grip on the steering wheel, or if they can't turn their head to look behind them because of neck pain.

    Driving a motorcycle is particularly problematic because you must bend the wrist every time you accelerate.

- **Public transportation.** Taking public transportation challenges RSIers, because if a bus or train is crowded, you must hold a pole as you stand. Holding a package, briefcase, or purse can be problematic too because of the strain on the hands and because, if you trip, you may not stop yourself from falling.

    Plan your schedule so that you do not use mass transit at peak hours, and sit in the seats reserved for people with disabilities.

- **Self-defense.** The hand is usually the first line of defense against aggression, and it eventually occurs to RSIers that if someone attacked them, they would be unable to defend themselves. Obviously, avoiding dangerous situations is prudent. Some self-defense schools teach methods of fighting with your feet.

- **Crowds.** If you experience excruciating pain when you are touched, you should avoid being in crowds where you might be jostled or bumped.

times miracles seem to happen—especially to motivated people who do everything they can to help themselves.

RSI SYMPTOMS RESPOND TO STRESS

Juliette Liesenfeld observed that her hands are magnets for stress. While riding in the car with her daughter, another driver came too close, and she felt the panic reaction in her hands. "With some people, it goes to the stomach; with me, it goes straight to my hands."

Stress flows along the path of least resistance to any area that is injured or weak. Such awareness can be useful (see box on page 56).

MEN AND WOMEN HAVE DIFFERENT RESPONSES TO RSI

RSI has affected many more women than men, but as men do more repetitive work, such as computing, the incidence of RSI among them begins to rise.

Men are at risk for severe injury if they respond to injury by trying to tough it out instead of seeking medical treatment. "To many men, the need to visit a physician is an indication of weakness and a devaluation of their masculinity," reports *A Man's Guide to Coping with Disability* by Resources for Rehabilitation.

While women are more likely to seek medical help than men, they run the risk of being dismissed by doctors as hysterical or hypochondriacal instead of having their condition treated. Changes such as pregnancy and menopause can also affect RSI, and many women say they experience greater pain around the time of their periods. This may be because of increased levels of certain hormones.

3

INJURY AND HEALING

To understand the recovery process, it is helpful to know how cumulative trauma injuries occur. By reviewing the factors that contribute to injury, we can better understand how interconnected the bodily systems are and why it is so important to have a total body health regimen to ensure that natural healing mechanisms function properly.

The Elements of Injury

SEDENTARY BEHAVIOR

According to the *Surgeon General's Report on Physical Activity and Health*, published in 1996, only about 15 percent of American adults perform twenty minutes of vigorous physical activity three times a week. About 25 percent of adults get no physical activity in their leisure time. In addition to contributing to the incidence of coronary heart disease, such sedentary behavior compounds the risks and severity of RSI.

You need a lot of upper-body strength and stamina to withstand the rigors of one common work task, computing. Just holding your hands to the keyboard for prolonged periods can be exhausting, which is probably why most people think it feels so comfortable to rest their wrist and forearms while they type.

A lot of people presume that because they get up and walk around frequently they are protected from RSI. But if you have bad posture and walk around with your head forward, shoulders slumped, and belly hanging out because your muscles are too weak to hold you in proper alignment, you are still at risk for injury.

POOR POSTURE

Good posture is the cornerstone for efficient muscle movement and is critical for the proper functioning of many activities, such as breathing and speaking. It is unfortunate that our society has moved away from insisting on proper postural training in children, because these habits are difficult to change later in life, especially if chronically tight muscles have altered bone alignment.

Working in a seated posture for prolonged periods is dangerous in and of itself. When performing tasks that require fine motor coordination, most people work in a head-forward position. Chronically tensing the neck muscles to support the heavy head weakens them.

Then there is the arm position. An average arm can weigh in excess of twenty pounds; just holding it extended for long periods, as you do for computer work, exhausts the muscles. Ideally, the arm's weight is distributed through the muscles of the upper shoulder and scapulae (shoulder blades). If the pectoralis (chest) muscles are tight, they can cause the shoulder blades to wing out from the rib cage instead of lying flush with it. Weak muscles between the shoulder blades, which could otherwise hold the wings in place, also contribute to this problem. Tight, shortened pectoralis muscles also can bind the nerves in the brachial plexus, leading to numbness and weakness in the arms.

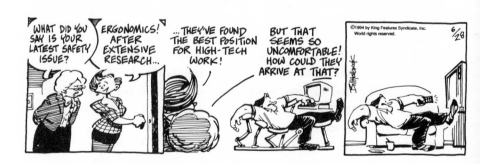

The forward shoulder posture also shifts the arm's weight to the upper shoulder and neck muscles, as Mary Lou Langford, an Albuquerque physical therapist, pointed out. "This stress can worsen the effects caused by the forward head posture, causing ischemia [localized loss of blood flow to the tissue] and pain in the chronically overworked muscles."

All of this is compounded by a bad chair. If people do not have proper seating, their bodies assume the dimensions of their furniture. Now the unnatural and strained posture of the capital letter "C" feels "normal," while good posture is difficult to achieve or maintain for more than a few moments at a time. To reverse these chronic changes or prevent further misalignment requires a combination of long-term soft tissue remodeling and postural retraining— plus a heavy dose of motivation. (See chapter 7 for more on posture.)

STATIC LOADING

"Static loading" is a medical term that refers to holding still while contracting muscles. This fatigues the muscles. An example of static loading is clutching a mouse while staring motionless at the monitor.

AWKWARD POSITIONING

The phrase "awkward positioning"—a favorite among ergonomists—is troublesome, not that it isn't a legitimate risk factor for RSI, but because most laypeople don't know exactly what it means. The human body, especially the hand and arm, has an enormous range of motion. The ability to *make* a certain movement does not mean it is safe to sustain or repeat it for prolonged periods. In fact, if you must sustain a position, proper positioning (with bones and tendons in neutral alignment) becomes crucial for safety.

The prolonged strain of static loading can make certain positions quite dangerous over time. Painting a ceiling, looking into a microscope, and extracting a tooth are all examples of awkward positions.

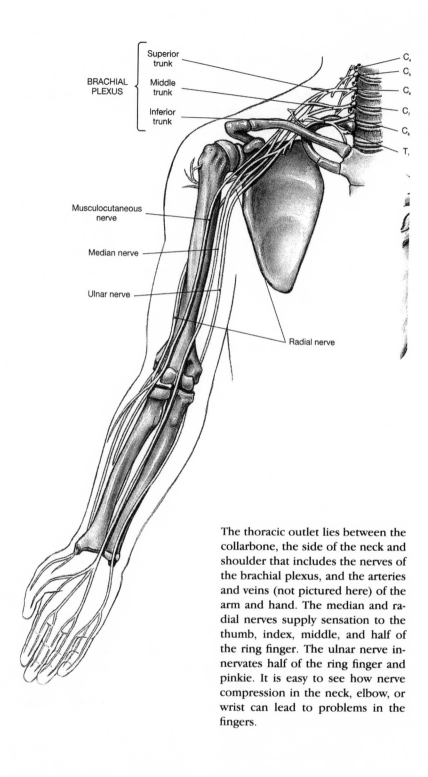

BRACHIAL PLEXUS

Superior trunk

Middle trunk

Inferior trunk

C₄
C₅
C₆
C₇
C₈
T₁

Musculocutaneous nerve

Median nerve

Ulnar nerve

Radial nerve

The thoracic outlet lies between the collarbone, the side of the neck and shoulder that includes the nerves of the brachial plexus, and the arteries and veins (not pictured here) of the arm and hand. The median and radial nerves supply sensation to the thumb, index, middle, and half of the ring finger. The ulnar nerve innervates half of the ring finger and pinkie. It is easy to see how nerve compression in the neck, elbow, or wrist can lead to problems in the fingers.

SITTING IS DANGEROUS TO YOUR HEALTH

While sitting is the most frequent body posture in industrialized nations, unfortunately, it is probably also the unhealthiest of all the prolonged postures, as Dennis Zacharkow notes in his book *Posture: Sitting, Standing, Chair Design & Exercise.* Sitting for prolonged periods is a huge risk factor for RSI, because this can combine static loading with improper posture. Most people do not know how to sit properly—with spine erect, as though standing—so they cave in to the confines of their chairs, which is a disaster if the chair is not properly designed.

Sedentary behavior—especially when combined with small-muscle gymnastics such as computing—is extremely hard on your hands and upper body. The head and torso are held virtually motionless for hours on end, but the forearms, hands, and fingers are running the equivalent of an eight-hour marathon. "It's not laying bricks, but it's comparable, given the muscles you're using," said John Cianca, M.D., a Baylor College of Medicine physiatrist.

In addition to the stresses of static loading, holding awkward postures such as the bent-elbow, palms-down position of computing are inherently dangerous. Nerves are stretched taut around bones, which can irritate them.

Sitting is also a significant risk factor because of what you are *not* doing. If you are sitting, you are not moving very much; therefore your blood does not circulate adequately, and you are not breathing as deeply as you would be if you were standing tall and walking.

IMPROPER TECHNIQUE

"Technique" refers to how a movement is performed. For instance, your computer technique would be how you habitually position your hands at the keyboard. Without realizing it, many computer users repeatedly misuse their hands at the keyboard or mouse, making themselves vulnerable to injury. Forcibly gripping a tool, whether it be a calligraphy pen or a hammer, is also poor technique and can lead to injury.

Learning how to position one's hands to ensure optimum alignment of the joints can reduce strain and the potential for injury. (See chapter 11 for more on technique.)

SPEED AND REPETITION

Once, during a lecture, a woman complained about how slow voice-activated software programs are. She wanted to know if there were any faster systems. Both of her arms were splinted to the elbow, yet despite her injuries, it had not occurred to her that her voice could sustain injuries from constant use as surely as her hands had.

One of the most difficult lessons RSI teaches is that the body is not meant to perform constant high-speed or repetitive movements indefinitely. The more frequently you make an awkward movement, the greater the stress to the soft tissue. This is particularly undesirable with small-muscle movements.

We need to respect the natural rhythms of life, now fast, now slow, now a steady pace. We also must respect the body's need to work as a whole instead of just the hands or only the voice.

FORCE

Using excessive force contributes to RSI by overloading the muscles. Examples of this include gripping a mouse and pounding a keyboard.

LONG HOURS

Despite all of our laborsaving devices, people are working longer and harder than ever. This means more repetition and muscle fatigue and less recovery time.

Computer users often think that they do not work long enough for it to be a problem. That may be true in a few isolated cases, but most people become so absorbed in their program they have no idea how much time they really spend computing; in fact, they spend much more time at the computer than they realize. Some people have become severely injured in relatively short amounts of time. One man said he wished someone would get rid of the myth that you have to work eight hours a day to sustain an injury. "I got injured, and I never spent more than two hours a day or forty minutes at a time using the computer." When he made these comments, he could not turn the pages of a magazine.

People tend to underestimate the time they spend at their computer. A businessman who spent several hours working at his computer in the office liked to play computer games after work to unwind. He said he generally played until one o'clock in the morning. "*Two* o'clock!" his wife interjected sharply.

ANATOMY

People readily accept that tall people can make good basketball players, beefy people can make good football players, and small people can be excellent gymnasts.

Yet when it comes to jobs that require repetitive fine motor skills, we do not seem to recognize that some people will do better than others in this regard based on their anatomical makeup. Muscle mass, flexibility, physical condition, and body type can vary significantly from person to person. Even nerve configuration, bone proportion, and muscle fiber composition can differ among humans.

COLD HANDS

Dr. Markison regards warm- and cool-handed patients as two distinct populations. Warm-handed people have enough blood flow to do well in recovery, assuming some behavioral changes are made, he said, but the prognosis is poorer for cool-handed people.

The tendency toward having cool hands can be related to stress. The fight-or-flight response originated with our evolutionary ancestors. When they were in danger, the blood drew away from their upper limbs to supply the brain, the heart, the lungs, and lower limbs, so they could flee. Office workers may not face saber-toothed tigers, but they may have a dragon of a boss, so the same reaction occurs today.

Cold hands often reflect poor circulation. If the blood does not reach the fingers, it cannot refresh the tissue with nourishment or remove metabolic debris. Cold slows the blood flow by narrowing the diameter of blood vessels. (See page 86 for hand-warming techniques.)

STRESS

In her study *Stress, health, job satisfaction,* Marianne Frankenhaeuser made an important distinction between negative and positive stress reactions. Human beings, she noted, can plan for the future, predict the consequences of certain actions, and choose between alternative strategies for problem solving. "When this capacity takes us through difficult situations, 'happy' stress predominates," she maintained. When we have a very demanding job but exercise control and influence over the work—as orchestra conductors do—stress can serve as a stimulus to make our talents flourish. Negative stress comes into play when we are not allowed any choice but must passively accept an aggravating situation.

Another problem associated with high stress levels is the lack of mobility, as shown in a study by Robert DeMatteo, Margaret Denton, and Lynda Hayward. The authors found that the more frequently workers could walk around and vary hand and arm positions, the less likely they were to report experiencing musculoskeletal symptoms. "Thirty percent of those who could not walk around reported 6 or more musculoskeletal symptoms compared to 2 percent of those who could frequently walk around," said the authors.

The modern workplace imprisons many people in what amounts to invisible straitjackets. Their heads are frozen forward, eyes riveted to the screen. The hands are shackled together at the keyboard. Some people won't even look away from their screen for fear that others will think they are not working.

BOREDOM AND LEARNED HELPLESSNESS

In modern work, much physical stress has been replaced by mental stressors, such as boredom. "It is time to kill the myth that pleasant and satisfying leisure can compensate for a boring, monotonous job," wrote Frankenhaeuser. "Work that kills initiative, insight and influence often makes us passive even during leisure—a kind of learned helplessness." This condition may develop in people who have been deprived of personal control over a long period of time. As Frankenhaeuser explained, "It does not pay to try, hence one remains passive even if the opportunity for change occurs. Helplessness once learned is difficult to overcome. Moreover, it tends to spread from one situation to another. "Work casts a shadow over leisure time. Stress hormones, heart rate and blood pressure remain at high levels."

TOBACCO AND ALCOHOL

Cigarette smoking increases your risk for developing RSI because it slows circulation. A study by Greek researchers found that the flexibility of the aorta, which transports blood to all parts of the body except the lungs, deteriorates as soon as one minute after smoking commences, and that this effect lasts at least twenty minutes after smoking. Smoking also decreases the flow of oxygen to tissues.

Consumption of alcoholic beverages—beneficial claims to the functioning of the heart notwithstanding—requires prudent monitoring. Overconsumption can damage general health and can affect the course of RSI.

IGNORING WARNING SIGNS OF INJURY

Some people wait until RSI has reached a crisis stage before they seek medical treatment. Other people seek treatment, then refuse to follow their doctor's advice to slow down or take time off work. Do not be complacent about RSI. If you have sustained an injury, you are at greater risk for reinjury, which can be more devastating than your initial bout.

The Elements of Healing

The body has great healing potential. Many severely injured people make great strides by patiently adhering to a health-enhancing lifestyle. Do not underestimate the power of these natural mechanisms.

REST

Rest is critical to healing, especially in the acute stage of injury. Resting does not mean complete inactivity; rather, it means ceasing activities that aggravate symptoms. So if you have a computer-related injury, you should also avoid other hand-intensive tasks such as sewing, carpentry, or playing musical instruments.

MOVEMENT

Movement is very healing to the body, because it stimulates the creation of synovial fluid, which bathes the joints and tendon sheaths. It also helps blood circulate and keeps muscles supple and strong. While aerobic exercise is necessary to keep the heart healthy, you need not work out violently or excessively to achieve results. Gentle movement such as brisk walking is enough to get your heart pumping, exercising your muscles and lungs.

CIRCULATION

Blood performs many important roles, such as nourishing soft tissues with oxygen and nutrients, and carrying away metabolites, the waste products of activity. Exercise and movement ensure that blood circulates through the body.

Blood volume is also important, because low blood volume results in higher concentrations of metabolites. Be sure to drink enough water over the course of the day to ensure adequate blood volume.

BREATHING

Proper breathing ensures that muscles are supplied with oxygen, which they need to function properly. Shallow breathing due to poor posture contributes to muscle tension in the neck, because instead of using your diaphragm, you use the muscles that lift the top of the rib cage. If these muscles become chronically tight, they can compress the complex network of nerves, arteries, and veins that squeeze under the clavicle (collarbone) on their way down the arm. Such compression can lead to problems such as thoracic outlet syndrome.

When you look at pictures of early typists, they sit nice and tall with straight back and neck. You rarely see anyone in a modern office adopt this position. Most of the time, we lean forward to read or write, with our spines and necks curved. Unfortunately, working hunched over a desk impairs the movement of the lungs and diaphragm, which are now prevented from fully expanding. It also constricts the abdominal and thoracic cavities, increasing the pressure on abdominal organs, which can impair digestion.

WARMTH

Because of the adverse effects of having cold hands, maintaining proper body heat is important. Some offices are kept very cold to protect the computer equipment; if this is the case, wear sweaters and loose-fitting fingerless gloves to keep hands warm. (See page 86 for hand-warming techniques.)

NERVES

Nerves send impulses and directives from the brain to distant limbs. Dr. Markison compared the process of nerve injury to stripping away the insulation of wire. Pain limits movement, so "when the nerve is unhappy, the hand stiffens up," he noted.

The process of nerve regeneration is quite slow and irregular. Warming hands, gentle stretching, and good posture may help sooth tingling nerves. Your doctor should also look for other conditions that may contribute to tingling, such as diabetes or a hypothyroid condition.

THE HEALING DIET

Patient: *Opening a bag of potato chips takes more effort than it used to.*

Doctor: *Other than potato chips, what do you eat?*

Food is the fuel of life. Despite the hundreds of thousands of dollars Americans spend buying vitamin tablets each year, there is no replacement for eating well. Food contains essential nutrients that are not contained in supplements, as well as fiber.

Food can also be medicinal. Take advantage of the natural anti-inflammatory properties existing in foods that contain omega-3 fatty acids, such as salmon, sardines, and tuna, and vitamin E, such as vegetable oils, leafy green vegetables, and whole-grain cereals. Antioxidant vitamins—C, E, and beta-carotene—help repair cell membranes. Rich sources of vitamin C include citrus fruits, broccoli, and cantaloupe; for carotenoids, eat dark green leafy vegetables (spinach is a good choice) and orange-colored foods such as carrots, apricots, and mangoes.

Approximately 55 to 65 percent of your diet should be carbohydrates (found in beans, whole wheat bread, and cereals); 20 to 30 percent fat (from sources such as olive or canola oil rather than animal fat); and 15 to 20 percent protein (obtained from fish, eggs, dairy products, poultry, meat, and tofu). Avoid high-protein diets. Too much protein can overwork your kidneys. As with excess carbohydrates, calories from unused protein are stored as fat. In addition, if your diet focuses on protein, you may not be consuming enough fiber or phytochemicals, important nutrients contained in plants, warned Susan Karp, who teaches nutrition at Marymount Manhattan College in New York. While phytochemicals have no nutritional value in the traditional sense, researchers are investigating their possible protective effect on the heart and potential anticancer properties.

Eat a diet rich in fruit, beans, and vegetables. The body is a moist medium, explained Dr. Markison. If you eat dry goods, such as fast foods, you waste body fluid and dehydrate yourself during digestion; whereas moist vegetable produce is relatively easy on the intestines. Further, studies by the National Cancer Institute show that people who eat lots of fruits, vegetables, and grains have enhanced disease resistance. Meat and other animal products are high in uric acid, which can lead to joint inflammation such as gout. "Meat should be a side dish, not the center of a meal," advised Karp. Soy products such as tofu are an excellent and healthful meat substitute.

Avoid high amounts of sugar, salt, and saturated fat (i.e., fat that is solid at room temperature), which can contribute to clogged blood vessels and impair circulation. One typical fast food meal, such as a hamburger, french fries, and a milk shake, could contain your entire day's allotment of fat—and a good number of your recommended calories. You should also avoid *trans*-fatty acids, which act like saturated fat in the body. These are listed as "partially hydrogenated" fats, and are commonly found in prepared foods, such as cereals, margarine, and baked goods.

Poor dietary habits, such as eating close to bedtime and consuming spicy or acidic foods, can contribute to vocal problems, too. "The stomach acid can actually etch the tissue of the vocal cords," said John Haskell, a speech pathologist and adjunct faculty member at Columbia University. This could contribute to the risks of injury associated with using voice-activated software.

Students of nutrition quickly learn that vitamin supplements cannot compete with Mother Nature in terms of how easily nutrients are absorbed. Furthermore, whole foods contain a wealth of vitamins and minerals and valuable compounds such as phytochemicals; supplements contain only one ingredient. Finally, supplements may be unnecessary and are potentially dangerous in high amounts, as in the case of vitamin B_6, whereas with food you do not risk overdosing (see box on page 38). Before you take supplements, ask a competent physician or qualified nutritionist about how to get adequate amounts of these nutrients through your diet. If you need supplements, ask for guidance in the proper dosage.

The best way to ensure adequate nutrition is to cook for yourself. Choose unsaturated fats such as olive or canola oil. Search for the freshest produce, and limit the amount of salt, sugar, and fat your meal contains.

Here RSI complicates matters; many people are too injured to cook. However, you can purchase low-fat, low-salt frozen meals and prechopped vegetables. When dining out, order heart-healthy meals, ask for salad dressing on the side, and have your food broiled or baked instead of fried. Shop carefully, because when you are hungry, you'll eat whatever is on hand. Your body replaces cells every day, and what you consume provides the raw material for new tissue, so use the best ingredients.

Eating well will help you maintain an appropriate body weight

Vitamin B₆

In recent years, vitamin B$_6$ has been promoted as a "cure" for carpal tunnel syndrome. However, you should be extremely cautious about taking supplements of this vitamin, because unlike some other water-soluble vitamins, B$_6$ can be stored in the muscles, and can thus reach toxic levels. Paradoxically, an excess of vitamin B$_6$ can lead to the very symptom people had hoped to relieve by taking supplements: nerve damage, which manifests as clumsiness or numbness in the hands or feet.

The Recommended Dietary Allowances (RDA) for vitamin B$_6$ are 1.6 milligrams for women and 2 milligrams for men. Significant dietary sources of this nutrient include: bananas, spinach, broccoli, tomatoes, whole grains, and beans.

According to the *Tufts University Diet & Nutrition Letter*, daily doses of 200 milligrams can be damaging to the nervous system. Yet vitamin B$_6$ is sold in doses as high as 500 milligrams—25,000 times the RDA—which an RSIer might unwittingly purchase in an attempt to help herself heal.

and allow your metabolism to be more efficient. One man quipped that RSI can be a great diet aid: He lost weight because it hurt too much to open the refrigerator door!

SLEEP

Sleep is another natural healing system. Unfortunately, worry and pain often keep RSIers up at night, or prevent them from getting restful sleep. If this is the case for you, try biofeedback or study self-relaxation techniques, yoga, or meditation. Sleep-inducing drugs are not recommended except for short periods under a doctor's supervision.

PAIN CONTROL

Heeding your body's warning signals helps; pushing through pain makes matters worse. Become aware of what you are feeling so you can respond to your body's subtlest cue. Learn pain control techniques such as the relaxation exercises taught in yoga classes or biofeedback, *after* you have sought medical advice about what is causing the pain.

AVOID SETTING DEADLINES FOR HEALING

Many RSIers often give themselves deadlines: "I have to be better in nine months because my concert tour begins then," a musician might say.

But deadline-oriented thinking can be dangerous. What if you are better but not strong enough to play an arduous program? Will you sacrifice months of painstaking rehabilitation for an evening program? Relapses are discouraging. Worse, pushing yourself beyond your limits can sometimes turn a moderate injury into a severe one.

Your body needs to recover on its own time, not according to the timetable you have set for it. This lack of responsiveness to the body's needs is part of what gives people RSI in the first place.

Instead, be patient and give your body all the time and attention it needs.

PACING

Although some people tend to drive themselves, most people would probably work at a healthier stop-and-start pace if left to their own devices.

"Pacing" means dividing the work into manageable loads, then stopping when you feel fatigue or symptomatic by either taking a break or calling it a day. It also means setting reasonable goals for the amount of work produced on any given day. If you experience pain or soreness, lower your workload.

Most RSIers are astonished at how long it takes to heal. "Two and a half months seems like eternity to you, but you get better in months and years," said Dr. Markison. "I've never seen anyone in the long term in exactly the same place year after year, five, six, or ten years into it. A patient I saw this morning was far better than she was four years ago. She doesn't even remember how bad she was. But I did, when I looked at my notes. You never know how much you can heal. That's the beauty of living. You have no clue as to where you're going to be in a number of years. You have to be supple, ready, flexible, receptive, welcoming and then you're fine."

4

THE EMOTIONAL ASPECTS OF RSI

Even people with the sunniest personalities can be shaken to the core when their hands give out. When she was diagnosed with RSI, Ellen K. said she felt as though her arm had "had a heart attack." Neill Rosenfeld burst into tears when his doctor told him to stop writing. After living with RSI for several years, Fran K. remarked, "It's just so hard being in pain every day. Maybe that's why I'm so cranky all the time."

Emotional angst often goes hand in hand with chronic disability and daily reminders of how life has changed. "You go to do something normal, and there are constant interruptions," said Ellen K. "If every fourth thought is being distracted, it's like Chinese water torture, drip, drip, drip. A friend showed me a new book, and I thought, 'Will I be able to turn the pages! Oh, what a beautiful object! Will I drop it?' "

The emotional state can mirror the physical stages of RSI; newly diagnosed RSIers' emotions are often as inflamed as their tendons. And as the physical symptoms of repetitive strain injury wax and wane, so too do people's emotional reactions to their injuries. You may find that there are days when you feel happy and hopeful, and other days when you feel as if you're being sucked into a black hole. Despite emotional tides, even severely injured people have found emotional equanimity after their diagnosis.

People with any illness will naturally try to find similarities and patterns to help them understand their situation. So it is not surprising that the idea of an "RSI personality" has been bandied about.

However, there are many reasons why this is not so. First of all,

RSI happens to laid-back people as well as driven perfectionists and all personality types in between. RSI can result from many kinds of overuse, including pleasurable pursuits such as playing tennis or golf. And RSI has many risk factors, including ignorance, lack of kinesthetic awareness, and anatomical predispositions. So while certain traits such as eagerness to please can be an additional risk factor for RSI, personality does not cause RSI.

Dr. Robert Rosenthal is a San Francisco Bay Area psychiatrist who treats people with chronic pain on a regular basis. He does not believe that the notion of an RSI personality serves RSIers well, for a couple of reasons: "The danger . . . is that you make an artificial distinction between those who have RSI and those who don't. It also adds the element of shame, because now, in addition to RSI, people have something *else* wrong with them—their personality, as if it were not just your body, it's who you are that made this happen. If you weren't that way, you wouldn't have RSI.

"What RSI people do have in common is that they overused their hands, and there may be personality traits that drove them to do that. [These traits might arise from parental pressure to base your self-esteem on work and achievement, for instance.] But I don't buy the concept of an RSI personality. It's essentially blaming the victim." Furthermore, an injury can have more to do with corporate culture and production quotas than an individual's personality.

Common Emotional Repercussions

SECOND-STAGE DENIAL

Even after accepting that you have RSI—and it's not going away— you may have trouble believing that your condition can worsen.

Jane H. did not take her doctor's advice to quit her job, for instance. "Looking back six years, I didn't think permanent disability could happen. I thought my eyes were wide open. I thought, 'This can't happen. I've overcome too much, too many obstacles in life, to lose my career.' "

Even changing the way she used her hands in daily life was a slow process for Jane. "I thought, those other people have to make changes, but I don't have to," she recalled. "I was still writing Christmas cards. I only recently agreed to use paper plates. I should have bought a telephone headset three years ago."

ANGER

People often become extremely angry when they realize they have lost normal use of their hands. This is perfectly understandable. However, anger tends to worsen symptoms, make you miserable, and alienate others.

Unfortunately, anger can be devilishly difficult to quell. Letting go of anger quickly—rather than replaying situations over and over in your head—helps. So does relaxation. (See box on page 56 and the discussion of relaxation in chapter 6.)

DEPRESSION

In some ways, emotional pain can be more difficult to bear than physical pain. Bleak moods can fairly blot the sun from the sky. Depression settles like invisible film over life, removing luster and joy from things once loved. It saps spirit and energy, and you feel as if it will never end. Depressed people often drive away the very source of comfort: other people.

Depression is a tricky topic when it comes to RSI, because we have a chicken-and-egg problem. Were you depressed before RSI, or did the injury trigger the depression? Regardless of which came first, it is important to take depression seriously, because it can have tragic consequences. Some people may find relief in psychotherapy; others may need antidepressant drugs for a time. Depression is treatable. You do not have to remain miserable, so seek help.

SUICIDAL THOUGHTS

Suicidal urges always arise from a sense of hopelessness. "Hopelessness is a symptom of depression," said Dr. Rosenthal. "It will go away when the depression lifts, either through antidepressant medication or psychotherapy."

Sadly, suicide among RSIers is not unknown. "The worst case was not my own [patient] . . . a teenager hung himself because of a diagnosis of bilateral carpal tunnel syndrome. He was obviously not aware—maybe not in touch with reality—that it was treatable," said Dr. Markison. "He killed himself. He was nineteen."

If you feel suicidal, please reach out to someone who wants to help you, either your own psychotherapist or a suicide prevention hotline, which is usually listed in the telephone book under "Community Services," "Crisis Intervention," or "Suicide Prevention." These services can sometimes refer you to a psychotherapist. Other sources of help are ministers, priests, rabbis, and trusted friends. When seeking a person to confide in, a good question to ask is: Who always makes you feel better when you talk to her?

If someone jokes about RSI ("I'd kill myself, but I'm too weak to pull the trigger"), be aware that this person may actually be thinking about suicide. Always take it seriously if someone threatens suicide, and suggest professional help. If you are upset by someone else's emotions, seek professional counseling yourself, as well as advice about dealing with the other person.

FEAR AND ANXIETY

Repetitive strain injury is terrifying in a lot of ways. Not only do people lose the use of their hands, which is a big contributor to feelings of powerlessness; they also face the terror of financial ruin. Relationships sometimes suffer because of an RSIer's depression or inability to carry out previous responsibilities.

One RSIer felt paralyzed with fear because she had a big project to finish—and after that, she did not know what she would do. No career paths felt right to her, and she was acutely aware that there would be a large gap in her life after the project was completed. "I feel like I'm going off a cliff," she said. Among other things, she feared how not being able to keep current with computer technology would affect her future career opportunities.

Fear can freeze the wheels of success while anxiety burns energy and erodes inner peace. Making concrete plans helps assuage anxiety.

GUILT AND SELF-RECRIMINATION

People with RSI may feel guilty when they no longer can volunteer to help with extra work or spend long hours perfecting a project. They feel bad if they do not rush to help with the dishes during family gatherings or fail to hold open a door for someone else.

However, in order to protect your recovery, you must avoid activities that trigger relapses. Decline with brief explanations, such as:

- "I'm sorry, I can't hold the door; I hurt my arm!"—preferably with a quick smile.
- "Would you mind getting that door for me? I'm afraid I can't manage it."
- "I'd love to help you move, but I can't. Maybe there's something else I can do." Then suggest something, such as watching the truck.

If you were sitting in a wheelchair, people would not expect you to get up and walk. But repetitive strain injury is a hidden disability. Your arms look fine to other people, so often they don't understand why simple things like carrying groceries, driving, or chopping carrots might be hard for you.

Depending on your personality, there are many ways to decline activities you know you should not do. For some people, invoking a higher authority is useful: You can say, "I can't do that—doctor's orders."

GUILT VERSUS SHAME

Psychiatry differentiates between shame and guilt as follows: With guilt, the feeling translates to "I did something bad," whereas with shame, it is "I *am* bad." If your inability to perform as you used to makes you feel unworthy or unacceptable, or you have an uneasy sense of being flawed or defective, this is probably shame.

"The cure for shame is gradually exposing what we thought was shameful in a safe setting—talking to a close friend, a support group, or a psychotherapist," said Dr. Rosenthal. "Discovering that others can accept our feelings and are not put off by them as we expected can be very healing of shame."

GRIEVING THE LOSSES OF RSI

Loss and limitation are actually part of the aging process. If we live long enough, we are likely to develop one infirmity or other, and some degree of diminished strength and physical ability.

RSI thrusts this knowledge on many of us at a relatively young age. It is not only possible but imperative to find another way to fulfill yourself or replace what you have lost. It can also be very helpful to do a little of what you love (see pages 54 [box] and 59).

Every case of RSI is unique, and everyone experiences loss in a different way. For Fran K., the loss of tactility was worse than the pain. "I have constant numbness. It feels like my skin is too tight or has things running under it. I can feel the ends of my fingertips, but there is a barrier between me and the object I'm touching. It's almost like wearing gloves, trying to feel through them.

"I get a lot of information about the world through my sense of touch," Fran explained. "The first thing I do is feel something. Doctors think if I can feel it when they test me with an instrument, that must mean I'm fine. Yes, I can feel, but it is not the same as gross motor coordination or touch. It is sort of like a musician losing part of her hearing. Yes, I can hear, but not the nuances."

For April S., an injured artist, the loss of work she loved was difficult. "I miss working with my hands," she said. "It calms me down; it's my therapy. It's not a hobby; it's a burning desire."

Bob Hubbard, an oboist, had a slightly different take on this situation. He, too, loves his work. "Playing music is a team sport like no other," he said. "It's a transcendent experience: You can lose your identity and become part of the flow. You're aware of your own part, but instead of planning the next difficult part, the mechanics disappear."

However, considering his long, satisfying career, he also knows "the overwhelming burden of doing it right all the time." Now Bob looks back "with nostalgia rather than loss."

Mourning this loss can be painful, but it is the first step in letting it go so you can start something new.

"My biggest disappointment was my friends," said April S. "I feel very alone. In social events, there are a lot of things I can't do. A friend wanted help painting her apartment, and I couldn't." Participating in sports was daunting, too. "I tried to jog, and it hurt my hands," she said.

RSI makes many people feel isolated from others. But having RSI helps you learn who your true friends are, and gives you the opportunity to form strong bonds with new people. Examine the basis of your friendships. "There are a lot of people whose friendships aren't very deep," observed Dr. Rosenthal. "If a relationship was based solely on playing handball every week, forget it. If the relationship were based on intimacy, which means you feel safe revealing your inmost self to another, it will survive."

Internet, Video, and Computer Game Addiction

Addiction to playing computer games or surfing the Internet is a serious emotional threat to healing. Kimberly S. Young, an assistant professor of psychology at the University of Pittsburgh, surveyed 496 heavy Internet users. According to her criteria, 396 qualified as on-line addicts.

Criteria included: staying on-line longer than you intended, calling in sick to work or skipping classes to use the Internet, experiencing withdrawal symptoms (increased depression, moodiness, or anxiety) when you go off-line, continuing to use the Internet despite recurrent problems it creates in your life, and making several unsuccessful attempts to cut down on the amount of time you spend on the Internet.

Denial can be a big factor in injury if someone cannot stop gaming or surfing even when experiencing pain.

Interacting with Other People

A host of activities uninjured people take for granted are difficult, dangerous, or impossible for RSIers. What you say about your injury—if you mention it at all—will depend on the situation. It is a good idea to practice using concise phrases to get the help you need without being sidetracked into long discussions about RSI (see box on page 52).

(see box on page 52).

ASKING FOR HELP

For healthy adults who have been accustomed to independence, being unable to do simple things can be a blow to their pride. "I don't like asking people for help," Kate M. confessed. "It's embarrassing."

In the early stages of injury, people often push themselves to do things they shouldn't do, but eventually they learn to ask for assistance. "The pain forced me," said April S.

Another way to approach asking for help is to reciprocate whenever you can. Ellen K. made several phone calls for European neighbors whose English was not good. "They asked how they could repay me." So she told them she would ask for their help if she needed to move some furniture.

FRIENDS AND SIGNIFICANT OTHERS

RSI can be trying for a friendship for a number of reasons. Your friends may become uncomfortable hearing about your disability because they are powerless to help you. Ellen K. said a friend finally confessed, "It hurts me so much to see you have this problem."

Your friends may be impatient for you to get well because they want the best for you. "I have one friend who keeps saying, 'Why don't you have the surgery? I just hate to see you like this,' " said Ellen. But in Ellen's case, as in so many others, there is no surgical remedy for her problem.

Some of your friends and relatives may not understand the depth of your problems. This lack of understanding can be very frustrating. During a long period of financial instability, Wendy F. confessed her difficulties to a friend, who replied, "Why don't you get one of those computer jobs on Wall Street? You could make a lot of money doing that!" Wendy's friend was delighted with her solution, until Wendy reminded her that she had been injured at the computer and could not do that kind of work anymore. "My friend knew quite well that I had RSI," she said. "I had repeatedly warned her about how disabling it could be, yet the reality of not being able to use your hands had not sunk in."

April S. had a similar experience. One friend who was trying to help her offered to pay her to clean his apartment. When April replied that she couldn't clean her *own* apartment, he became angry.

Sometimes noninjured people become so overwhelmed by their inability to help you that they cannot bear to hear you talk about coping with this disease. "They say, 'Oh, it's terrible—I can't talk about it.' *You* can't talk about it!" April continued. "When people say, 'Maybe the injury was meant to be,' I could kill them."

Many healthy people do not understand what it means to have a chronic problem. Said Wendy, "My boyfriend asked what I had done one day, and when I told him, he said, 'You sure have a lot of doctor's appointments,' as though I were a hypochondriac."

Another woman complained that she was tired of having to ask her boyfriend for assistance. "I finally said to him, 'Why don't you offer to help me? You can see this is hard for me.' " Her experience saddened her. "It says something about the relationship," she observed. "My best friend is not like that at all. She says, 'Let me get the door; let me do that for you.' She's right inside my head."

Minimizing conversation about your injury is useful, because unless people have RSI, they generally cannot understand how much it limits you. You don't want to be perceived as a whiner or be treated like an invalid, so keep the focus off your disability as much as possible.

PEOPLE WHO PUT THE BLAME ON YOU

He jests at scars that never felt a wound.
—WILLIAM SHAKESPEARE, *Romeo and Juliet*

Lynette C. had an experience that is not uncommon. An acquaintance insinuated that Lynette's RSI resulted from her own specific weakness, instead of being something that could happen to anyone. Sometimes people start asking pointed questions about exactly what kind of work you were doing, or what computer program you were using, or how long you worked. The purpose of this avenue

In Defense of Etiquette

True etiquette involves showing kindness and consideration toward one's fellow human beings. It is not about being a snob or using the right fork. Good manners can be of great benefit when talking about RSI.

For instance, while some RSIers are delighted to discuss their symptoms, surgeries, and travails, others would prefer to be more private about their medical history. Good manners require that strangers refrain from prying into your health status beyond a polite "How are you?" Concerned people will wait until you initiate the topic or give you an easy-to-escape query such as "Is there anything you would like me to know?" (To which you might respond, "Thank you so much for asking, but no" or, "Thank you, yes"—and then get whatever it is you want to say off your chest.)

If you are sensitive about discussing your medical condition, you will probably appreciate such tact. Some people, however, seem to have gotten through childhood without being taught that it is rude to press on with inquiries even when those questioned become visibly ill at ease, reply in monosyllables, or attempt to change the subject. This unfortunate trend toward no-holds-barred questioning has not been helped by tell-all books and talk shows.

of inquiry, said Dr. Rosenthal, is "to find where you are at fault so they know it couldn't happen to them."

You can handle this situation by saying that the risk factors for RSI are quite variable, but your doctor assured you that it could happen to anyone who has used a computer.

ACQUAINTANCES

It is usually a good practice not to bring up your limitations with acquaintances unless you absolutely have to. If you are meeting someone for a fleeting moment, it may be better to minimize your situation. If you are in a situation where you must ask for help, keep your requests and reasons brief and matter-of-fact. Say, "Can you help me with this? I hurt my hands."

TALK TO PROFESSIONALS

When you have serious problems, there is nothing worse than well-meaning people offering simpleminded advice. It is also hurtful to have them dismiss your problems because of their own ignorance.

Talk to people who can help you: other RSIers who maintain a positive outlook, and understanding physical therapists or psychotherapists. That way, you can vent your feelings in a safe manner rather than compounding an insensitive remark by getting upset about it.

Steps to Emotional Healing

If you are very depressed or having trouble coping with other feelings, seek the counsel of a professional psychiatrist, psychologist, or social worker right away. These people are trained to offer help in ways that friends and loved ones sometimes cannot. Don't let financial constraints stop you from getting valuable advice. Ask a social worker for a referral to a low-cost or free clinic. In some states, Workers' Compensation might cover psychotherapy, especially if your depression arose in response to your injury.

Even if you are not in particular emotional distress, here are eight strategies for maintaining a good outlook throughout your RSI recovery process:

EXPRESSING EMOTIONS SAFELY

Despite the current emphasis on controlling emotions, we are not meant to be unfeeling beings. Emotions are meant to be expressed. "I don't like the word 'control,' because it implies there is some-

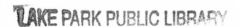
LAKE PARK PUBLIC LIBRARY

Sample Script

Practicing graceful ways to say no or seek help is very important. Here is a sample letter or speech you could adapt for friends, coworkers, and associates. Use words that are comfortable for you, and practice saying them until they roll off your tongue. The more comfortable you are with your condition, the more you will put others at ease, and the more likely it is they will help you.

Repetitive strain injury is a serious disease, which is frequently the result of overuse of the hand. It can happen to anyone who does repetitive work. RSI damages soft tissue, such as nerve, tendon, and muscle. Sometimes, as in my case, this can go on for years.

My doctor and physical therapist have told me how to take care of myself. I am not supposed to strain my hands. Certain activities—or doing too much of them—can worsen my condition. Simple actions such as turning a doorknob or pressing an elevator button may be easy for you, but because of my injury, those things can cause excruciating pain to me.

My symptoms fluctuate, so some days I can do more than others, and some days less. Just because I am not feeling acute pain does not mean my injury is cured. To maintain my recovery, I need to respect my physical limitations. I am doing everything I can to get better, and I am deeply grateful for your patience and understanding. Believe me, if I could use my hands normally, I would.

thing wrong with your emotions," observed Dr. Rosenthal. Instead of trying to "control" or stifle your feelings, talk them over with a friend or therapist. If there is something you can change, take action and this will help you feel better. If not, accepting your life as it is and seeking inner serenity may be the key.

"We want to communicate so someone understands how we're feeling," said Dr. Rosenthal. "But there is a difference between expressing your emotions and battering someone with them. Battering is inflicting your emotional state on somebody else—that's not communicating."

HAVE A GOOD CRY

"There are times when I go home and I have a good cry and that's enough," said Kate M. "Sometimes all the bad days can press into one and crying doesn't help."

A good cry can be a cleansing outlet for emotions. But if you find that you are crying very often or uncontrollably, get professional counseling.

AVOID ISOLATION

We all need warmth and companionship. Many RSIers who lose their jobs become very isolated. They spend hours at home alone, with little to distract them from pain and fear. This can lead to a downward spiral of despair and depression.

"Some people are so lonely it's scary," said Sylvie Erb, a New York physical therapist. "They tell me they keep the TV on all day so when they come home they will have a presence there."

This is when an RSI group can literally be a lifesaver. Bonds form with other people in the group; friendships are made. If you know that certain people are depressed, you can call to chat with them and let them know how important they are to you, even if they might secretly feel worthless now that they can't make a contribution at work. If you are feeling vulnerable one day, another RSIer might be thrilled to hear from you, never mind that you feel down. By giving and receiving emotional support, you can keep one another afloat through difficult times.

Some people are shy about asking for help; but remember, it can be a joy to feel that you have helped another person.

Groups serve all kinds of purposes. They can be sources of referrals, resources, support, and a place where loaded emotions can be discharged. However, it can be very upsetting if group members habitually explode in rage. "Emotions are contagious," noted Dr. Rosenthal. "Anger is particularly dangerous because other people may mirror that. While it is important for people to tell their story, if a group ends up magnifying anger, that's not going to be useful to anyone. But if it helps soothe, gives people a safe place to express anger, that is healing."

Doing What He Loves, One Minute at a Time

The amazing story of Jimmy Amadie, a jazz pianist, appeared in *Keyboard* magazine. His struggle with RSI testifies both to the time and patience it takes to heal, and to the power of the human will to triumph over difficult circumstances.

As a young musician, he would play two hours of Bach, two hours of Beethoven, two hours of Mozart, two hours of Chopin. Then he would warm up for two more hours. "After that, I'd do the gig. And after that, I'd show someone how fast I could play octaves."

After several years, Amadie first experienced hand discomfort, then pain, until one night, "I raised my hands, I hit the keyboard, and both of my index fingers collapsed. That was it. I lost everything. I was out of the business."

Amadie suffered agonizing pain for years. He consulted thirty-five doctors in three years and underwent two surgeries. He taught and wrote for his living.

If you are forming a group, you might consider having special meetings for members who want to focus on positive things. An atmosphere of peace, trust, and serenity helps the healing process. Try not to complain, because that generally escalates feelings of anger.

SURROUND YOURSELF WITH POSITIVE PEOPLE

Have you ever noticed how relaxed you are in one person's presence? Or, conversely, how upset you feel around someone else?

Choose upbeat, easygoing companions whenever possible. When you must be around someone with a negative attitude, such as a family member, limit your time together. Spending time around

> When he tried to play, the pain came back. After a hiatus of seven years, Amadie began a program of recovery. He allowed himself one minute per day of careful practice. Six days later, he had such agony that he was forced to quit for a month. Amadie persisted. He worked back up to playing a minute each day, increasing three minutes per day each year. Eventually, he could play twelve minutes a day.
>
> Amadie agreed to play with Dizzie Gillespie, Buddy Rich, and an all-star band. To prepare for the performance, he doubled his time. "By the sixth week, I couldn't lift my arms or get out of bed. Once again, I couldn't play. I couldn't even do my minute a day."
>
> Amadie had further surgery and began anew. He re-weighted his piano keys and set up a home recording studio. Little by little, he planned to record an album, in painstakingly slow segments. "None of them will go for more than eight minutes; I don't want to blow my chops again. But for that eight minutes, man, I can play with anybody."

positive people can take your mind off your own problems. Although an RSI support group can be a wonderful source of support, do not limit yourself to fellow sufferers. Keep in touch with former colleagues and associations.

TRAIN YOURSELF TO BE AN OPTIMIST

Many people do not realize what a potent tool optimism can be. On an unconscious level, we respond to how others perceive us. So if we radiate confidence and good cheer, others will reinforce those feelings.

Even if you weren't born an optimist, you can train yourself to be one. As with strengthening exercises for the body, you do not see results right away, but if you are faithful about your regimen, eventually you will achieve your goal. Essentially, it boils down to changing how you think about things. Whenever you find yourself getting worried, angry, or frustrated, consciously replace negative thoughts with positive ones. It's as simple—and as difficult—as that!

Emotion-Washing Technique

When strong emotions such as anger or fear come up, allow these feelings to "wash" through you. For instance, if you feel forearm pain in response to a strong feeling, immediately relax and imagine the pain traveling out your fingertips. Concentrate on getting your breathing back to normal as quickly as you can. By shedding the feelings as quickly as possible, they will not get the chance to settle into your soft tissue.

This trick works amazingly well even in periods of great stress. It will be easier to use if you also practice relaxation techniques or meditation.

PRACTICE POSITIVE SELF-TALK

How you talk to yourself about your situation can make a big difference. When Lynette C. was going through a difficult period with her RSI, she repeated over and over, "I don't deserve this. I'm a good person, and I've worked hard, and I deserve better." Her mantra helped her maintain her self-esteem and avoid self-defeating behavior.

REFUSE TO BE A VICTIM

As difficult as living with RSI is, if you whine and complain about your fate, you will be perceived as a victim and people will avoid you. "People hate victims, because it makes them feel victimized," said Rebecca Chalker, a health writer. "They feel pulled into it."

There's a big difference between presenting yourself as a person with a disability and as a disabled person. Do not act like a victim. Instead, be the triumphant survivor you are.

TAKE CHARGE

Learning how to control your pain and taking action to get your life back on track will be emotionally healing. Taking care of yourself is better than always depending on someone else to make you feel better, because then you are in control.

Small Ways to Save Your Sanity

QUALITY-OF-LIFE CHOICES

Sometimes solutions seem obvious—unless you haven't thought of them yet. A friend of mine told me how he handled depression a few years ago. "I got so tired of that New York in-your-face attitude," he said. "I like it when people say 'Please' and 'Thank you.' So I decided that when I bought my coffee and bagel in the morning, I would go to the *nice* place. I wouldn't go to the place where people shouted 'Next!' or didn't say 'Hello' and just stared at me."

Gary's Story

Gary Karp is a San Francisco–based ergonomics consultant. He is currently writing a book titled Life on Wheels, *an overview of the wheelchair experience.*

People are usually surprised when I tell them that I have experienced myself more disabled through the RSI than through my paralysis. I was eighteen years old when I was injured. I fell out of a tree and had a spinal cord injury. Not being able to walk was something that I could adapt to pretty easily. It seems like such a big thing, but the fact is you develop the strength in your arms. You learn certain skills. Wheelchairs are getting better and better all the time. Employment, transportation, and public facilities are improving and social attitudes are adjusting, so the paralysis is actually a manageable disability, at least in terms of being as active as I want to be. I got an education, I had a job, I traveled, I did pretty much what anybody else would—and more, in a lot of cases.

The RSI is another story, because all of a sudden, my ability to control my mobility became a factor. I didn't want to make a change to a power wheelchair,

Quality-of-life issues add up after a while, so look at ways you can increase the chances of having pleasant interactions in your own life.

THE THERAPEUTIC VALUE OF WORK

Work can distract you from pain, giving value and meaning to your life, and remind you that you still count as a person. Whether you are paid for it or not, be sure you have a project that you enjoy.

because when you do that, then you're not using your body.

I was in a company for nine years. I was a manager, I had respect and authority and was well paid, but it was a very stressful type of life. The relationship that I had with one of the owners was increasingly strained, because he was not good at sharing power. Anybody in the history of the company ultimately would leave as they rose up through the ranks, because nobody could partner with him.

I got caught up in trying to prove myself to the owner of my company. I felt threatened by the fact that he was sort of pushing me aside. He didn't want me to proceed with passion and pursue ideas that I had for the company. My makeup is to bang harder at it, trying to prove myself, which implies a certain amount of self-doubt. I was working so hard, trying to compensate for other dynamics. If I injured myself, then obviously something was out of balance. RSI was a message.

I didn't work for a year during my Workers' Comp disability period. Then I made a decision that I was going to do ergonomics, speaking, and consulting. As a result of my injury, I have a new career, and a woman who called me as a client became the love of my life!

DO A *LITTLE* BIT

Completely giving up a beloved activity may not be entirely necessary. As Gary Karp, a skilled guitarist and juggler, noted: "It's not easy to let go of doing the things that you love. I'm not willing to say I'm never going to do those things again."

Talk to your doctor and physical therapist about hand-intensive activities. It may be okay to do a *little* bit. But read about Jimmy Amadie to learn what a little bit means.

TREAT YOURSELF THE WAY YOU WISH
OTHER PEOPLE WOULD

Sometimes it helps to imagine that you and your symptoms are two different people: You are the parent, and the pain is the child. Wise parents know impatience makes things go more slowly, whereas tasks borne with patience proceed apace; and praise often works better than condemnation. So if you allow yourself to become frustrated with a slow recovery, you bring an added pressure to an already burdensome situation. Be as gentle with your symptoms as you would be with a beloved child.

CULTIVATE A WINNING ATTITUDE

Your attitude can make or break your recovery. Even a surgery patient's feeling toward her stitches can be revealing, noted Dr. Markison. "You've got a choice. It's either horrible that you've had your body opened up to have some tissue rearranged, or you can look at the stitches and say, 'Well, that looks nice.' Then it's an ornament—as opposed to something ghastly."

MAKE AN EFFORT

In this culture, people sometimes attribute success to luck, talent, or privilege. Even when successful people cite hard work and dogged perseverance as the primary source of their good fortune, luck—not effort—is seen as the major factor.

Effort will get you farther with RSI than any lucky breaks. Doing your exercises, keeping a positive attitude, and maintaining patience over the long haul will pay off.

MIND OVER MATTER

While there may not be a definitive cure for RSI and other serious diseases, embracing a healthful lifestyle and understanding the source of painful feelings can help symptoms subside, if not disappear altogether.

"I do believe symptoms can go away if you resolve the underlying emotional conflict," said Dr. Rosenthal. He still hears from a patient who recovered from reflex sympathetic dysfunction—an extremely painful and debilitating condition—this way.

5

MEDICAL TREATMENTS

Though overuse injuries were described in the early 1700s by Bernardino Ramazzini, known as the "Father of Occupational Medicine," many aspects of treatment—from resting, avoiding strain, and performing only gentle exercise—remain the same. Thus far, modern medicine has not come up with a quick cure for many soft tissue injuries, so people must instead cultivate patience as Nature does her slow work.

Overview of Current Treatments

RSI is frequently treated in ways that are actually counterproductive to healing. For instance, a doctor will prescribe a splint, which can lead to further weakness and injury if not done judiciously. Doctors also commonly prescribe anti-inflammatory medications, which unfortunately do not cure problems arising from a bad workstation and often do not help with the symptoms of RSI, either. Anti-inflammatory drugs can have serious side effects (see page 65). The same is true of repeated cortisone injections, which can weaken muscle tissue and lead to scarring. Nor does surgery always bring the desired outcome of eliminating pain and regaining hand function.

Exercise should focus on strengthening the muscles of the mid- and upper back, not those of the forearm or hand, which typically have been injured from overuse. Unfortunately, some physical therapists have people squeezing rubber balls and doing wrist curls—which can aggravate an injury.

Lessons from Medical History

"It seems extraordinary how little of wisdom of the 19th century was passed on to the 20th," lamented Hunter Fry, an Australian surgeon, in an article on overuse injuries in musicians. Indeed, many of the observations made a century ago by G. V. Poore, a physician, are as true today as they were then. In the quotes that follow, he was speaking of musicians, but his comments—published between 1887 and 1899—apply to many other occupations as well.

ON REST:
The most important point in treatment is rest. The excessive use of the hand must be discontinued, and it is often necessary to insist upon this rather forcibly.

The Proper RSI Examination

A thorough RSI examination can take an hour and a half, because muscles, nerves, and posture must all be evaluated.

HISTORY AND MEASUREMENTS

Your physician should take a complete occupational medical history, and ask about other medical conditions such as diabetes, arthritis, and thyroid disease. Your height, weight, hand dominance, and hand temperature should be noted. Your hand-grip and finger-pinch strength should be measured. Some doctors measure the circumference of your upper arms and forearms to see if any atrophy has occurred. Previous injuries to the upper extremity should be noted. Active and passive range of motion of the neck, shoulder,

ON OVERWORK:

It is often difficult to restrain the ardor of these patients in the matter of playing. Directly they feel in a small degree better, they fly to the piano; and I have known the progress of more than one case very seriously retarded by the undoing, as it were, of the good effect of rest by an hour's injudicious and prohibited "practicing."

ON IMPROPER EXERCISE:

Patients often think that their ills are to be cured by gymnastics, such as the use of dumb-bells and the like; such a proceeding cannot do good, and, if the muscles be overstrained, may do harm. I always discountenance any kind of violent exercise with the arms, and recommend any gentle exercise which involves no prolonged strain, and does not cause pain, stiffness, or uneasiness. There is no object to be attained by keeping the arm and hand in a sling (which I have frequently known to be recommended); there is no reason why the patient should be deterred from making ordinary use of the limb.

elbows, forearms, wrists, thumbs, and fingers should be measured. Signs of swelling should be noted.

POSTURE

A thorough doctor will look for postural problems, such as a forward head, protracted shoulders, or one shoulder high or low. If any of these problems exist, postural retraining and soft tissue manipulation may be prescribed.

NERVE TESTING

There are a number of tests for nerve compression. Your doctor may press deeply into certain trigger points at the thoracic outlet (near the neck by the collarbone) or tap lightly on the elbow and wrist to see if you experience pain or other symptoms. (See glossary under *Semmes-Weinstein Monofilament Test*, page 215.)

PALPATION

Your physician will press your muscles to see if they are tender, or run her fingers along a tendon to see if it feels grainy. Muscle tightness can also be determined this way.

NECK

To test the movement in your neck, you may be requested to turn your head from side to side (as in shaking your head no) to see if the movement is symmetrical, and tilt it up and down (as in nodding yes) to observe the range of motion. Sometimes X rays will be prescribed to note the presence of an extra rib, joint degeneration, or other bony conditions.

SHOULDERS

Your doctor should have you raise your arms to the front, side, and overhead to determine whether you have good range of motion. You will also try to touch your hands together in back as though scratching between your shoulder blades.

ELBOWS AND FOREARMS

Your physician may perform this common strength test: You bend your elbow and resist him while he pulls your forearm down.

WRISTS

Your doctor may ask you to move your wrist up and down to measure its range of motion.

FINGERS AND THUMBS

You will make finger movements, such as touching the tips of your fingers to your thumb, reaching your thumb to the base of your little finger, or making an "O" with your thumb and index finger while the doctor tries to pull them apart. Your doctor may press down on your fingers and ask you to push up, or use other strength-testing procedures.

FOLLOW-UP CARE

Once your doctor has examined you thoroughly, she will often prescribe physical or occupational therapy or other treatments, which are described later in this chapter. You may be instructed to rest the inflamed area and then begin a slow rehabilitation routine of strengthening exercises and gentle stretches to regain range of motion. Massage and physical therapy can be very useful.

Your doctor may also write a note to your employer about your needs for special equipment, self-pacing, and home treatment (such as ice for pain). If you are troubled emotionally by your injury, your doctor may refer you for psychological counseling or tell you about local RSI support groups. Many physicians are able to advise their patients about Social Security Disability and other avenues of help.

Your doctor may refer you to a specialist for further testing or to a surgeon to see if surgery is indicated. A thorough exam usually includes a follow-up appointment so that your doctor can see how you are progressing. Ideally, the physician will also be in touch with your physical therapist and will advise you on workstation modifications and special equipment, such as telephone headsets.

Drug Therapy

Physicians frequently prescribe nonsteroidal anti-inflammatory drugs (NSAIDs) for RSI. These can include: Anaprox, Butazolidin, Fenoprofen, Indocin, Motrin, Nalfon, Nuprin, Tolectin, and Voltaren. Such drugs can have serious side effects, notably abdominal cramps, ulcers, sunburn, flulike symptoms, or, in rare cases, anaphylaxis, an allergic reaction. If you have symptoms of anaphylaxis,

Dr. Piligian's Patient Recovery Checklist

Here is a checklist Dr. Piligian uses to make sure he has thought about the various aspects involved in caring for a patient with RSI over the long term. Not every physician will have the ability or the resources to address all of these needs, but you can seek further qualified assistance to fill in the gaps for yourself, using the suggestions in this book (see Resources, page 223).

☐ Prescribe physical or occupational therapy as needed.

☐ Prescribe postural or movement retraining as needed.

☐ Advise about strength training, flexibility, and aerobic exercise needed.

such as a rapid pulse, fast breathing, swelling around the eye, or fainting, have someone drive you to the emergency room immediately or call an ambulance and wait for it with your feet elevated higher than your head.

Ask your pharmacist for advice on how to take these medications, and for possible drug interactions.

As an alternative, ice can be very effective in treating pain and inflammation. Talk to your doctor first, to see whether you have any conditions that would make the use of ice unwise, such as Raynaud's disease. Vitamin E, a natural anti-inflammatory, might also help; ask your doctor or nutritionist for the correct dosage. With vitamins, more is *not* better!

Low-dose antidepressant drugs such as Prozac, Zoloft, and Elavil are also used to treat the pain of RSI. No one quite understands how they work, but it could be that the medications prolong the

☐ Prescribe various pain-control and relaxation techniques, as needed. Instruct person about the importance of setting aside time during the day to use these interventions.

☐ Ask if the person suffers from depression, feels angry, or has other emotional issues. If so, refer for counseling, i.e., to a social worker or psychologist.

☐ Where relevant, suggest that the person tap into religious or spiritual beliefs as a source of comfort and healing.

☐ If the patient needs assistance with insurance matters, financial problems suffered from job loss, or finding help with legal matters, refer to a social worker who can make further referrals as appropriate.

☐ Advise about workstation adjustments. Write a note for employer if necessary.

☐ Suggest sources of further education about RSI.

☐ Make a follow-up appointment.

presence of serotonin, a chemical produced in nerve cells that attaches from one nerve ending to another. Sometimes heart medications such as Mexiletine, or antiseizure medications such as Tegretol, are prescribed as well.

TRIGGER POINT AND CORTISONE INJECTIONS

Trigger point injections of either saline solution or local anesthetic can help disrupt spasm and release the tight muscle to its proper length.

Cortisone injections are used to reduce pain and inflammation. This treatment should be used sparingly, however, because cortisone can weaken tissue and sometimes rupture tendons. "Injections work poorly for some reason in cool hands," noted Dr. Markison.

What to Consider About Surgery

Many people would like to avoid the knife at all costs, and in many types of RSI—typically muscle strain injuries—there are no surgical remedies. But surgery is sometimes necessary to treat carpal tunnel syndrome and other nerve compression syndromes. Surgery may also be necessary for severe constrictions of tendons, such as tennis elbow (epicondylitis) and De Quervain's disease, or removing a ganglion cyst. Surgery for thoracic outlet syndrome may involve removing an extra cervical rib or the first rib, or dividing the muscles above the collarbone. When facing surgery, choose the doctor with the greatest amount of experience and who has had good results with his operations.

Carpal tunnel surgery is performed two ways. In the carpal tunnel release, a small incision is made on the palm side of the hand, the ligament is divided, and when it grows back together there is more room for the median nerve. Dr. Markison compared it to unbuttoning a tight collar on a shirt.

This surgery is also performed with one or two small incisions parallel to the wrist crease. An endoscope cuts the ligament from below. An endoscope is a fiber-optic light and camera with a cutting instrument attached. The surgeon can view the procedure on a video monitor. Sometimes patients are able to heal more quickly and return to work sooner with this type of surgery. Dr. Markison says he tried the operation, but "I felt I wasn't seeing enough through the endoscope." He thinks there is more risk of an incomplete release with the endoscopic method, and prefers the minimal-incision open carpal tunnel surgery he performs. Postoperative care typically involves wearing a splint to protect the wound. Stitches usually come out in ten to fourteen days. Sometimes physical therapy is prescribed.

According to Dr. Markison, trigger finger operations can take fifteen minutes; carpal tunnel or ulnar nerve releases typically take

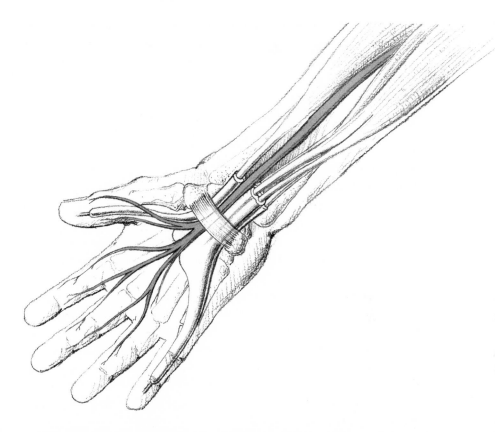

The transverse carpal ligament, or flexor retinaculum, forms the roof of the carpal tunnel and holds the median nerve, tendons, and synovial sheaths within the carpal tunnel. Tendon sheaths allow tendons to glide through a tight area. The basal thumb or carpometacarpal joint is vulnerable to overuse injuries from activities such as using a mouse and the space bar.

twenty to thirty minutes; radial or cubital tunnel surgeries can last 45 minutes to an hour; and a basal thumb joint reconstruction could take an hour to an hour and a half. Surgery performed under local anesthesia might cost $500; operations requiring general anesthesia could run $5,000 (including hospital, anesthesiology, nursing, and surgical fees). Recuperation can take from four to eight weeks. These estimates are approximate; discuss the particulars of your operation with your surgeon.

Whether to have surgery is a difficult decision for many RSIers, who may feel pressured by employers, insurers, and friends to have—or avoid—surgery. Decisions about surgery must be made on a case-by-case basis. Discuss the possible outcomes with your doctor. It is good practice to seek a second opinion if your doctor wants to perform surgery, but that is not the only time you might need to seek another physician's viewpoint. It is also a good idea if you get the impression your doctor does not understand RSI or does not take your complaints seriously, or if you feel you have not received a thorough diagnosis.

Types of Physical and Occupational Therapy

Physical and occupational therapy can help people control pain, improve range of motion, and build strength and endurance. Some doctors happily prescribe rehabilitation therapy; others do not seem to be in favor of it. A good rehabilitation therapist is worth her weight in gold. Take advantage of the opportunity to educate yourself and ask questions about self-care while you are in treatment.

In addition to hands-on treatment, such as deep tissue massage, physical therapists use a host of modalities to treat RSI. These can include hot and cold contrast baths and transcutaneous electrical nerve stimulation (TENS), which involves positioning electrodes on painful areas and sending a mild electrical current through them. In iontophoresis, creams containing cortisone or a conductive solution are rubbed on the skin, and an electrical stimulation device is moved over the cream, allowing it to penetrate through to the tissue to reduce inflammation. In phonophoresis, an ultrasound device is rubbed over conductive gel or cortisone cream; in ultrasound treatments, no medication is used. Some rehabilitation therapists use low-energy lasers (also called cold lasers) to stimulate circulation in the area. Therapists also evaluate posture and prescribe exercise.

If you find that one sort of treatment seems to work wonders for you but another does not seem to help, tell your therapist so she can focus on what benefits you most. If a modality does not help you in several weeks, it probably is not worth continuing.

A WORD ABOUT SPLINTS

Many doctors express dismay about the widespread prescription of splints for people with RSI. "The quick and simple solution to all this stuff is to drug them and splint them and send them away—and chide them that they don't make progress on that regimen," observed Dr. Markison. Dr. Piligian was horrified to learn that some companies were "passing splints out like candy." Splinting is a medical treatment and should be performed only under a doctor's supervision.

As Ann Barr pointed out, "Splints are used to immobilize acutely inflamed tissues during periods of rest. The splint should support the affected area in an anatomically 'neutral' position. Only in rare cases should splints be worn during dynamic activity. In these cases, specialized splints intended for this purpose should be customized for the individual patient."

If a resting splint is worn during activity, further injury may be produced in the injured and/or adjacent tissues. If there is swelling, "splints may further compromise circulation and fluid return, thereby paradoxically impeding healing," she continued. Splints may lead to disuse atrophy or contracture of immobilized tissues; therefore, it is important that they be used in conjunction with appropriate exercise.

There is another very good reason to avoid unnecessary splinting: "If you wear a splint," said Dr. Markison, "the world will give you advice about something they know nothing about."

HOW TO CHOOSE A REHABILITATION THERAPIST

Choosing a rehabilitation therapist is quite similar to choosing a physician. You can ask friends, other RSIers, and your doctor for referrals. Then ask yourself: Does she respond to your concerns? Does she teach you how to perform exercises properly? Does she answer your questions? Remember, no matter how high the recommendation, if you do not feel confident about your treatment, you should keep looking.

Because we are human, we respond differently to practitioners as well as treatments. Take the case of Gerrie G. When her physical therapist, whom we shall call Susie, went on vacation, Gerrie started seeing someone new. While working with Karen, the substitute, Gerrie made dramatic strides. She wanted to switch therapists, but hesitated because she did not want to hurt Susie's feelings.

After much deliberation, Gerrie eventually switched. Her choice did not reflect badly on Susie, whom many other patients found helpful. Gerrie was right to work with Karen, and free Susie to help those who respond better to her style. Professional physical therapists understand this sort of thing and are not upset by it.

WHEN TO CHANGE THERAPISTS

Though the majority of physical and occupational therapists adhere to the highest professional standards—and many of them are quite knowledgeable about treating RSI—a few RSIers have had unpleasant experiences with them. Their experiences are included here so that if you find yourself in similar circumstances, you will seek better treatment.

When April S. started physical therapy, she had no idea what to expect. She later described the experience as "dreadful."

"The therapist made me exercise with weights, very fast," said April. "When I complained, she said, 'That's the way we treat RSI.' I told her I didn't like it. My hands felt tired and sore. I had my appointments before work, and it took a half a day at work to recover from the exercises. I was really unhappy. They gave me a list of exercises, but I didn't know if I was doing them right or wrong.

"Now I know I did all the wrong things. I was angry with myself that I didn't listen to my intuition."

Another RSIer, Jane H., had a series of troubling experiences with physical therapists, too. When she was initially injured, she went to one facility, where the therapists discouraged her from entering the Workers' Compensation system, the appropriate choice since her injury was work-related. "They made nasty comments about people who used Workers' Comp. It was guerrilla tactics to get rid of Workers' Compensation patients."

She eventually went to another facility, and once again had problems with her physical therapist, whom we will call Jill. "Jill hurt me in a couple of ways. She didn't know much about RSI. She had me convinced I had no upper-body strength. She said she knew good exercises. I didn't have a problem doing exercises, because I've always been physically active."

But, as Jane found out, there is a right way to exercise—and a wrong way. "She was never satisfied. I'd say, 'Okay, Jill, I did a hundred reps.' But I never did good enough for her. She kept giving me more work. The weights were too heavy. There were too many reps. And she's not the kind of person you can escape. She would watch me. She was very critical."

Jane got married during this period, and she did not ease her routine even on her honeymoon. "Jill scared me so much I could not give up this aggressive work," she recalled. "You know how it is when you're in love? You just want to be with this guy. I tore myself from my husband to go to the gym. I would work out for two hours Monday and Wednesday, and for two to three hours Saturday." Though her routine seemed excessive, Jane remembered thinking, "Jill would know; she's the expert." But finally, she could not keep up. "My hands had curled up and they were ringing electricity. I could not hold on to a coin to put it into the slot. The very aggressive physical therapy program didn't work in the long run. I wound up working myself into the ground."

She went to her doctor, who urged her to quit her job. "I said 'No way.'" Jane switched doctors—and, once again, physical therapists. Once again, she got an overzealous physical therapist who pushed her hard. Now Jane performed two and a half hours of exercise every other day. "At the time, I didn't want to admit this whole thing isn't working and that my first doctor was right—that I should quit my job. So I threw myself back into the program."

She felt a little better for a while, then her condition deteriorated rapidly. "I left my job because I was in so much pain. I had trouble holding a fork."

Today, Jane is seeing a therapist who uses a gentler approach. "Now I'm doing ten important exercises and taking [an] extra-gentle yoga class for injured people. Maybe stopping the job, and doing slow stretching, will allow the body to heal itself," she said.

LENGTH OF TREATMENT

Physical and occupational therapists often provide an oasis of tranquillity for RSIers in distress. Because they see RSIers so frequently, they sometimes know better than anyone else the devastation RSI has wrought in patients' lives. Some grateful RSIers feel their physical therapists have saved their lives, in more ways than one.

While rehabilitation therapy can be very beneficial, many doctors and therapists worry about patients becoming overly dependent on them. Eventually, patients should learn enough about caring for themselves to leave extended treatment and begin self-care. Learning to take care of yourself becomes even more critical in managed-care settings, where the number of sessions you receive may be very limited.

However, it is troubling that many rehabilitation centers arbitrarily end treatment for RSIers. Sometimes health maintenance organizations will not deviate from an allotted number of sessions. "They kick you out whether it's better or not," complained one woman.

This kind of forced "graduation" can be meaningless in terms of real recovery. "Technically, I graduated—but I was in pain for four months and I lost my job five months later," Jane H. recalled. By discharging people before they have reached maximum recovery, these institutions in effect abandon their patients.

There may be several reasons for this. One rehabilitation therapist explained, "There has to be an end to treatment. If anyone pulled my files and saw how long I'd been seeing patients, I'd be so embarrassed!" Perhaps she felt those RSIers who failed to improve reflected poorly on her. But from these patients' point of view, her treatments—which helped them remain pain-free and function as well as possible—were enormously valuable. Perhaps if this important role received more acknowledgment, the rehabilitation therapist would feel differently about early termination.

Also, insurers frown on continuing to help people who may not be making much progress, using the argument that since these individuals are not improving, it is not worthwhile to continue treatment. Progress is sometimes subjective: From an RSIer's vantage point, relief from pain is a great benefit, especially when symptoms worsen once treatment ends.

Many physical therapists decry this situation. Ideally, the decision to leave physical therapy should be mutually acceptable to the patient, her doctor, and the physical therapist.

NEW THERAPIES

Regretfully, I cannot recommend any new breakthroughs at this point. Some RSIers have tried various treatments, but so far no one has been cured by them. One woman had laser treatments for carpal tunnel syndrome. At first she was excited that her hands felt almost normal for the first time in a long time. Several months later, she reported: "It seemed very promising in the beginning, but in the end it didn't help. I had a series of treatments, and on the last one, the doctor said, 'You're cured.' Even then I thought it was a joke—that he was trying to influence me psychologically, which didn't work."

She went back to see him when her symptoms got worse again. "He was surprised to see me. Maybe he really believed I had been cured. But if he counts me as cured, that's not right," she said.

Most health professionals think that RSI is too complex to be resolved by a single approach. At this point, the best treatment for RSI is embracing a healthful lifestyle, avoiding reinjury with prudent hand use, resting when needed, and patiently allowing Nature to do her work.

Relapse: The Second Wave

They keep finding new things wrong with me.
—KATE M., after a visit to her doctor

Having lived with RSI for many years now, and having watched many other RSIers cope, several phenomena that were not obvious in the beginning reveal themselves. This is purely a personal observation. To my knowledge, no one has studied the following paradox.

First, while there is always reason to hope for improvement, many people think that their RSI is "cured" after the initial bout of injury and rehabilitation therapy. Later, they notice that their hands become hypersensitive: They are susceptible to heat and cold or any kind of strain. During the initial stage of injury, Juliette Liesenfeld,

Osteopathy

In my opinion, osteopathy is the best-kept secret in Western medicine. Developed in 1874 by Andrew Taylor Still, this technique relies on hands-on manipulation of tissue to unblock areas of constriction and improve the circulatory and nervous system (but it should not be confused with chiropractic work). There are still a number of osteopathic physicians who practice in the traditional manner in the United States and Canada. However, as Andrew Weil noted, "Most contemporary D.O.s [osteopathic physicians] give drugs and recommend surgery just like their M.D. colleagues. Few of them use manipulation at all, and fewer still rely on it as a main modality of treatment."

Osteopathic practitioners believe that problems arise when natural movement is impaired, and once mobility is restored to tissues and joints, the body heals

a book translator, could still drive. Now, a year later, her hands have improved, but she cannot drive anymore. "It's paradoxical," she noted. "My hands were better when they were worse."

Other RSIers have expressed the same sentiment. "I thought it was worse last year, but this year I can do less," said Kate M. This hypersensitivity is probably due to scarring, muscle tightness, and lowered tolerance to stress and exercise.

Second, RSI does not always stop with the initial injury. Rather, physicians tend to find more and more maladies in RSIers as time goes on. "There is a chain reaction, which occurs as the result of compensatory adjustments to the underlying injury. It boils down to too much use with too little strength and endurance," explained Dr. Cianca.

itself. Some practitioners claim that the body is really doing all the work; they are merely helping that natural process along—and certainly never forcing things. "You *suggest* to the tissue; you don't impose," emphasized Philippe Druelle, D.O., founder of the Canadian College of Osteopathy in Toronto. Osteopathic practitioners look at the whole body instead of one isolated part. Ten men or women can complain of similar pain, but it may not necessarily stem from the same cause, noted Druelle.

Osteopathy has helped me in dramatic ways. Chronic neck pain all but vanished. Numbness and tingling diminished. Strength and endurance increased. Improvement has taken time, but has been well worth it, and the changes in my body have been lasting rather than transitory.

The best news about this work is that it is covered by insurance.

GETTING WORSE WHEN YOU'RE DOING ALL THE RIGHT THINGS

After my initial diagnosis of repetitive strain injury in 1991, I immediately embraced the things that would help me heal, and my condition improved. By faithfully following a strict regimen of physical therapy, strengthening exercises, proper computing technique, and careful pacing—plus a healthy dose of positive thinking—I did well for a couple of years. Acute pain greatly diminished. My grip strength increased by twenty pounds as a result of my exercise regimen. I still got sore easily, and so could not work at the computer for as many hours as before, but I was grateful to have as much use of my hands as I did.

But as time went on, my condition worsened despite my painstaking efforts. Two years after my initial injury of lateral and medial epicondylitis, thoracic outlet syndrome was diagnosed. Two years after that, cubital tunnel syndrome and the beginnings of carpal tunnel syndrome had been diagnosed.

In the spring of 1996, things took a sharp turn for the worse. I kept dropping things; I would wake up with numb hands; I had tingling during the day. When I went on vacation for ten days, there was barely a buzz, but upon coming home and writing by hand for an hour, my symptoms flared ferociously. It disturbed me that my endurance was so poor—I used to be able to work for four to six hours a day, but now I felt I was pushing things after forty minutes.

My experience is hardly unique. Many other people go through exactly the same pattern: They get an initial diagnosis for tendinitis in the wrist, for instance. But as time passes, they get thoracic outlet syndrome, cubital tunnel syndrome, or other ailments. Weakness and injury in one area often sets off a chain reaction of other injuries, like a row of dominoes collapsing one on top of another. After seeing this happen again and again, I started asking doctors why it occurs. When one area is hurt, people often get compensatory or substitution injuries.

Dr. Cianca explained the tendency toward reinjury as follows: "When you come out of the womb you're brand spanking new, and for a period of time you're just perfect, like any new car. But as you use your body more and more, it starts to show signs of age. Things wear down, and some structures don't work as well. When tissue is injured, it has had to repair itself—and that reparation is never as good as the original structure. As you get older, there's a natural attrition of muscle and other types of tissue, so you have less to work with. Injuries become more significant: Even if they do heal properly, you're dealing with less good tissue and more scarred tissue. Although you may be functional, you just may not be as smoothly functional as you once were."

In the worst-case scenario, according to Dr. Cianca, "you have to operate with some discomfort or some compensation for the way you used to do things. You never really get back to what you were before the injury. Now, it doesn't have to a big difference, but sometimes it is. I think that's the worst thing with people who have these repetitive use injuries. The more they have them, the less likely they are to go back to pain-free function."

After my initial diagnosis, like most people, I wanted to continue working at all costs. Much later, I realized I would probably have more use of my hands today had I stopped and rested instead of worked during my rehabilitation.

It seemed to me that the continued use of the computer was the culprit here. A review of the risk factors for RSI suddenly made more sense than ever, especially all the admonitions about static loading. People focus on repetitive *movements* as the only culprit for RSI. But holding still is equally bad. Just having your elbows bent for long periods can strain some nerves because of the prolonged stretch. I realized that the simple act of typing—even though I was not in acute pain—could in fact be reinjuring damaged tissue.

This is not to say that every case of RSI will turn into an endless series of relapses and further diagnoses. But it is all the more reason to carefully monitor how you use your hands every day.

6

COMPLEMENTARY AND SELF-CARE TREATMENTS

As Americans grow concerned about the side effects associated with many drugs or about surgeries going awry, more and more people are seeking alternative healing methods. "When people who don't feel well are told that they are well no matter how they feel, or who are given pills instead of good dietary or lifestyle advice, you create a gap in care that complementary medicine is rushing to fill," noted Michael Carlston, M.D., who teaches an elective course in homeopathy at the University of California at San Francisco. (Homeopathy, which means "similar to suffering," is a system of medicine that uses small amounts of substances that stimulate the same patterns of symptoms to trigger the body's healing mechanism, according to Dr. Carlston.) Indeed, according to Carlston, about 40 percent of all medical schools are offering courses in some aspect of alternative medicine.

Though some physicians are open-minded about—and even supportive of—these therapies, many patients feel compelled to seek treatment without telling their Western-trained physician.

There are two important points to keep in mind if you decide to use alternative therapies for RSI. First, be sure your doctor and rehabilitation therapist know you are using these techniques so if there is a potential problem you will be aware of it. Second, just because a treatment works for someone else does not mean it would be good for you. A friend might derive great benefits from acupuncture, for instance, but for you the results may be nil.

Remember, too, that no one approach will solve every problem of RSI. Acupuncture will not improve faulty typing technique, poor posture, or improper pacing. Massage will not get your heart pumping the way exercise will. Thinking positive needs to be reinforced with taking the right kinds of actions.

Take a synergistic approach.

Complementary Therapies

Most people with RSI try an array of treatments to help themselves heal. While Western medicine has much of value to offer, there are also many useful techniques that fall into the category of complementary medicine. Lots of RSIers choose to take advantage of both types of medicine.

Here are brief descriptions of some treatments for RSI—many of which I have personally found to be useful. This section is not meant to be all-inclusive, and it does not cover many commonly available methods that have been adequately dealt with in other publications. Just because a technique is included here does not necessarily guarantee it will be effective; it is mentioned because some RSIers have found it useful and you might, too.

Read through these descriptions, and if they appeal to you and you find them helpful, wonderful. Remember, though, your case of RSI is unique. Some people find massage highly beneficial, but if it causes you pain, you might want to try therapeutic touch or the Alexander technique. If the idea of acupuncture frightens you, try acupressure—which does not involve needles—instead. Biofeedback might help people who find meditation difficult. Find your own favorites and use those that help you best.

ACUPUNCTURE AND ACUPRESSURE

This ancient Chinese healing art has gained widespread acceptance in recent years; in fact, an increasing number of Western-trained physicians now treat patients with acupuncture. By delicately placing needles along certain acupuncture points, the chi, or body energy, is allowed to flow freely.

Having acupuncture bears no resemblance to having blood drawn or getting a shot. The needles are tiny and often barely penetrate the skin. Most acupuncturists use disposable needles to avoid the risk of infection.

In acupressure, the practitioner uses fingers—rather than needles—to release the points. Sometimes a point can be tender; if it is painful, the practitioner can hold the point longer rather than using deeper pressure.

Some people find acupuncture especially helpful for low energy, anxiety, and pain. The powerful pain-relieving quality of this work should not be abused, however: Do not feel you're entitled to overwork or push your hands just because they do not hurt.

HYPNOSIS AND SELF-HYPNOSIS

Contrary to what most people think, hypnosis does not mean that you hand your power over to another person, who can then make you do things you do not wish to do. Some doctors have found the use of imagery and suggestion useful in increasing hand warmth and reducing pain. Dr. Rosenthal sometimes tells patients to "close your eyes, relax, and imagine the feeling of your hand lying in the warm sun" as a way of raising hand temperature.

Dr. Markison also teaches patients self-hypnosis as long as they are comfortable with it. "If someone is afraid of bringing up repressed memories, it's not a good idea. If you are happy daydreaming, it will probably work for you. Otherwise it can be a mind minefield," cautioned Dr. Markison. Hypnosis is best done under the careful guidance of a credentialed psychotherapist or physician.

BIOFEEDBACK

Biofeedback was developed in the late 1960s by Joe Kamiya, a researcher who studied human consciousness at the Langley Porter Institute in San Francisco. Kamiya wanted to see if people could become aware of their brain activity and learn to control it using instruments that provide continuous information about muscle tension or brain waves by emitting a tone, light, or computer display. This process allows the person to gain control of blood flow, muscle tension, or brain waves.

Biofeedback can be very useful for improving posture, warming fingers and toes, pain control, and relaxation, according to Julie

Weiner, a biofeedback practitioner in Yonkers, New York. Electroencephalogram (EEG) biofeedback of certain brain wave patterns also appears to improve slow-wave sleep, during which the body produces growth hormone and repairs tissue.

THERAPEUTIC TOUCH

This gentle technique, developed by Dolores Kreiger and Dora Kunz in the 1970s, actually involves either very little or no touch. Rather, the practitioner—often a nurse—will work with the body's energy fields. If you observed a treatment, you would see the practitioner passing her hands inches above the recipient's body, often in long downward strokes. What effect could this have? you might wonder.

To find out, I had a treatment with Sue Duncan, a New York occupational health nurse who teaches therapeutic touch. Sue asked me to sit, then said, "Tell me if anything feels uncomfortable."

As Sue worked, I was aware of her hands though she rarely actually touched me—and then only with a few light strokes. Soon there were vivid reactions: Tension in my neck released, it felt as though the blood flow was stronger in my arms and legs, and my hands were warm as toast.

At one point, there was a nice sense of heaviness in my body; at another, it felt as though it were filled with helium. The treatment was deeply relaxing, and the effect continued as I rested afterward. My energy remained high through the remainder of the day and evening.

Therapeutic touch may be helpful to you if you find massage painful. It is simple to learn—perhaps you can trade treatments with friends.

THE ALEXANDER TECHNIQUE

This movement reeducation technique was founded by F. Matthias Alexander, an actor, in order to solve the vocal problems that were ruining his career.

With verbal imagery or guiding touch, students learn how to eliminate habits of bodily misuse—such as excessive neck tension or round shoulders—in simple activities such as sitting, standing, and walking. In addition to greater ease of movement, some students have found relief from chronic pain, stress reduction, improved breathing, and enhanced performance, according to Tom Vasiliades, an Alexander technique teacher in New York City. I tried an introductory session with Tom, during which he had me recline upon a table, then guided me through subtle movements with verbal instructions and light touch. The table work was particularly powerful for pain relief, and my posture felt naturally centered after the session.

Some people study this technique for years, but Vasiliades said you should have a basic understanding of it in ten to twenty sessions. He said he was initially attracted to the work because his teacher told him he could achieve the benefits of the technique on his own, not just with the assistance of a teacher.

MASSAGE

If you use a computer, or do any kind of close work, massage can be a good way to reduce stress, improve circulation, and maintain flexibility. Even when they are not injured, many people schedule massage once a week as general maintenance.

There are many types of massage—Swedish, shiatsu, neuromuscular, to name a few—and they can be quite distinct from one another. Sometimes doctors prescribe therapeutic massage, which may be covered by insurance; ask your physician for a prescription if you want to give it a try.

Massage need not be painful or deep to be effective. Tell your massage therapist about the kind of pressure you prefer, and about past injuries or sensitive areas. If massage hurts, let your massage therapist know. You do not have to endure anything that does not feel right to you. Massage techniques vary from practitioner to practitioner and from school to school, so if one method does not work, try another.

MYOFASCIAL RELEASE

Fascia is the glue of the body, enveloping muscle and other structures in a continuous sheet. If fascia hardens in one area, it can pull on areas both near and far from the original site. In myofascial release, the practitioner stretches the tissue using gentle, sustained pressure rather akin to pulling taffy. This can restore flexibility and release bound-down muscles to normal length.

Though subtle, this work can be powerfully effective in reducing pain.

Selecting What's Best for You

CHOOSING A PRACTITIONER

When choosing a practitioner, you're looking for the right mix of chemistry and competence. Find someone who makes you feel comfortable *and* helps you progress.

The level of skill among practitioners of healing therapies can vary quite a bit. Before you give up on an approach, consider trying someone else.

COMPARING THE COSTS

Alternative therapies tend to cost less than Western medical services; however, as the joke goes, they require alternative forms of payment because these charges are often not covered by medical insurance. More and more Western doctors are practicing acupuncture, and some doctors are happy to write prescriptions for complementary techniques such as biofeedback and massage. Talk to your doctor to see if there is a way your treatment can be covered by insurance.

ARE YOU READY TO HEAL?

Sometimes no method of healing—not even surgery—is successful if people are not ready to heal, health professionals have observed.

Possible roadblocks could be: using a disease to avoid having to assert your needs; needing love or attention; or believing that your illness is the only way to keep a significant relationship. Sometimes people hold on to pain as punishment for something they feel guilty about. If you suspect that is the case with you, discuss your ambivalence with a psychiatrist or psychologist so you can make the most of the healing opportunities available to you.

Self-Help Techniques

The idea of taking good care of your body is a sound one, because while doctors and rehabilitation therapists are valuable members of your recovery team, they can help you only up to a point. Much of your recovery will depend on you, because you are the one who uses your hands. Your doctor cannot sit up straight for you. Your physical therapist cannot do your exercises for you. Only you can practice patience and restraint, avoiding the things that will exacerbate your injury, doing the things that help you heal and remain stable in recovery.

There is a big difference between caring for your injury and treating it. Self-care encompasses things like pacing, avoiding activities that trigger symptoms, and doing your exercises. Self-treatment might mean taking high dosages of self-prescribed vitamins, or using home ultrasound devices, lasers, or other self-prescribed gadgets. In other words, self-care is doing what your doctor tells you to do, but treatment is the professional medical practitioner's job. Tools that are effective in the right hands can be dangerous if you are not properly trained to use them. If you have questions, ask your doctor or physical or occupational therapist for advice.

RSIers develop an arsenal of tricks to assuage pain. Ellen K. lies down if she is in great pain, because it is the only way she can relax her arm muscles. Others apply ice. I have found regular exercise—properly designed for my body and injuries—to be one of the best ways to stay pain-free.

Here are some other ideas.

HAND-WARMING TECHNIQUES

You can warm your hands either by raising your body temperature through exercise, biofeedback, or self-hypnosis, or by external means, such as bathing them in warm water.

Dr. Markison suggests that his patients have a glover make loose fingerless gloves from cotton spandex or polar fleece that cover the hand from the second knuckle to above the elbow to help hands retain warmth. If you cannot have gloves custom-made, cut the fingers from store-bought ones and wear long-sleeved shirts. If your gloves leave marks on your skin when you take them off, they are too tight. This interferes with circulation. Physical therapists can provide tube lining, which is not a glove but a comfortable stockinette that can be worn on the forearm and upper hand.

In cold weather, glove underliners are available through catalogs and sporting goods stores.

HERBAL REMEDIES

Dr. Markison tells a story about a patient who performed an experiment with herbs. "I want to show you something about healing from the plant world," she announced. She had had surgery on

---

The Breath Trick

This exercise is good for people who tend to breathe shallowly (which exacerbates thoracic outlet syndrome).

To get a sense of diaphragmatic breathing, lie on your back in a comfortable position on the floor (put a pillow under your knees if you have back problems; rest your elbows on pillows if need be). Place one hand above your belly button and the other on your sternum.

Now inhale through your nose and exhale through your mouth, and practice feeling the hand on the belly rise and fall with each breath, while keeping the chest and neck muscles perfectly quiet. This exercise goes quite nicely with the couch trick (see page 89).

the injured fingertips of both hands, and she applied aloe vera and goldenseal to one hand but left the other alone. The side with the herbal ointment healed faster.

Check with your own surgeon before using this method. Your doctor or physical therapist can also prescribe silicone gel packs to help soften scar tissue after surgery and might be able to recommend over-the-counter herbal preparations to soothe symptoms.

Healing Through Acceptance

"In our culture, we're trained to reflexively run from pain," said Dr. Rosenthal. "But I heard about a Native American tradition of touching the part you hurt with the object that hurt you. For example, if you stub your toe on the door, instead of shouting obscenities, bring your toe back and gently touch it to exactly that part of the door where it was injured. This promotes an attitude of acceptance."

Dr. Rosenthal used the power of acceptance to great effect: "I was cooking and accidentally cut myself deeply preparing Thanksgiving dinner. I got real calm and told my wife I needed to be by myself. I decided that even if I had to go to the emergency room, it would still be a good Thanksgiving—and I would have a scar to remind me of how well I handled this."

Not only did Dr. Rosenthal not need to go to the emergency room (he bandaged the wound himself), he reported that the pain was gone in ten minutes, and he never got a scar.

Obviously, as a physician, Dr. Rosenthal could gauge his need for emergency medical services. If you gash yourself, seek medical advice *and* try to make peace with the injury, if you choose.

THE COUCH TRICK

This is a great thing to do anytime you feel neck strain: Lie on your back on the floor, with your knees bent and your feet elevated on the couch. (A stack of pillows or a chair will work in a pinch.) Your thighs will form a right angle to your spine. Rest your elbows on pillows if it is more comfortable. Now just relax, letting your spine sink into the floor. You can either doze or practice diaphragmatic breathing in this position for as long as you like (see box on page 87). Be sure to support yourself carefully as you get up and down from the floor.

FLOTATION TANKS

Some RSIers, like Gary Karp, use flotation tanks for therapy. "They are good for stress reduction because you're suspended, and all muscular tension is relieved," he said. In addition, because you are isolated in the tank, your brain gets a rest from external stimuli.

If you float, remove your contact lenses first. You can leave the tank door open if you feel claustrophobic.

PILLOWS

It is very soothing to pile some big pillows on your lap and rest your arms with palms faceup. You can keep a pillow at work and also use this trick at home while viewing television or chatting with friends.

PAMPERING

While not a treatment for the hands per se, having a facial, mani-cure, or pedicure can be relaxing. And if you are the type of person who has trouble slowing down, it is a way of forcing yourself to get away from stressors and worries for a while.

PETS

Pets can offer practical, as well as psychological, comfort. Animals are marvelous listeners. They never offer unsolicited advice or make insensitive remarks. They are always happy to see you, no matter what kind of mood you are in. In addition to companionship and affection, dogs and cats can keep your hands warm while you pet them.

Dogs also provide built-in health benefits, since you will get regular exercise yourself by taking the pooch for a walk. If you have a dog, be sure it receives good obedience training. A forty-pound dog pulling on a leash can strain your hands; be sure it responds to voice commands.

Cultivate Ambidexterity

During a lecture at the Harvard Club in New York City, Dr. Markison remarked at one point that everyone should actively cultivate ambidexterity. "Why wait until the drill press crushes your dominant hand?" he asked.

At the time, his statement seemed rather zealous. Now it makes enormous sense. Anyone who injures the dominant hand instantly sees how very unwise overreliance on that hand is.

Dr. Markison suggests training the nondominant hand by using it to paint with watercolors, because you will most likely be less judgmental of your work this way. For excellent advice on how to begin, see Betty Edwards's *Drawing on the Right Side of the Brain.*

Be patient with your hand training. Think of how long it takes children to learn the complex act of handwriting. Begin slowly, when you are in an unhurried frame of mind. If you find yourself becoming frustrated, take a break and come back to it.

CHINESE IRON BALLS

In Chinese culture, rolling two iron balls in the palm of one's hand is said to promote health. You will instantly understand how this activity promotes dexterity, especially if you make the balls go counterclockwise. Truly skilled people never let the balls—which are sometimes filled with noisy chimes—touch.

To practice dexterity, try rolling the Chinese iron balls in your palms clock- and counterclockwise (unless you would aggravate an active inflammation in your hands or forearms by doing so). If the balls are too heavy, use two walnuts. James Wang, a New York physical therapist, said his grandfather used the same two walnuts for many years, until the oils from his hands burnished them to a rich, dark mahogany.

This practice is also thought to calm the mind, most likely because you cannot worry about problems and control the balls at the same time.

Relaxing Is Essential to Recovery

[P]eople are already suffering from stimulus overload. The nervous system evolved in low-stimulus environments, and many people still yearn for a return to that natural state of quiet and serenity. They'd rather take a walk in the woods than view "Gone with the Wind" on their wristwatches.
—GERALD W. GRUMET, responding to an article about multimedia in the *New York Times*

Relaxation is usually the farthest thing from your mind when you face the prospect of long-term disability and possible unemployment or when you are enraged at your boss, doctors, or the Workers' Compensation system. Yet the ability to relax is so critical to healing that Dr. Markison observed, "The only patients I've seen do really well with RSI have learned some sort of relaxation techniques."

Blood circulates more freely in relaxed muscles, warming limbs and carrying oxygen to distant tissue, then cleansing away waste products. This facilitates healing. Chronic muscle tension thwarts the healing process.

The Relaxation Workshop: A Blueprint for Healing

WEEK ONE: BREAKING THE CYCLE OF STRESS

Constant stress is a poor environment for healing. The Relaxation Workshop emerged from an observation that the ability to relax is the first step in healing; after all, what good is "rest" if your muscles

Wanted: Equal Education

Ben Franklin wrote the following essay on ambidexterity in 1785:

**A PETITION TO THOSE WHO HAVE
THE SUPERINTENDENCY OF EDUCATION**

I address myself to all the friends of youth, and conjure them to direct their compassionate regard to my unhappy fate, in order to remove the prejudices of which I am the victim. There are twin sisters of us; and the two eyes of man do not more resemble, nor are capable of being upon better terms with each other than my sister and myself, were it not for the partiality of our parents, who made the most injurious distinction between us. From my infancy I have been led to consider my sister as being of a more elevated rank. I was suffered to grow up without the least instruction while nothing was spared in her education. She had masters to teach her writing, drawing, music and other accomplishments; but if, by chance, I touched a pencil, a pen, or a needle, I was bitterly rebuked; and more than once I have been beaten for being awkward, and wanting a graceful manner. It is true, my sister associated with me upon some occasions; but she always

are tense from worry and fretting? RSIers needed a place where they could get away from their worries for a while and relax. Nothing that took RSIers' special needs into account existed, so I designed the Relaxation Workshop. The goal was to interrupt the cycle of worry/stress/pain/worry, and allow the healing process to begin.

In the first session, the goal is to consciously relax here and made a point of taking the lead, calling upon me only from necessity, or to figure by her side.

But conceive not, sirs, that my complaints are instigated merely by vanity. No; my uneasiness is occasioned by an object much more serious. It is the practice of our family that the whole business of providing for its subsistence falls upon my sister and myself. If any indisposition should attack my sister—and I mention it in confidence, upon this occasion, that she is subject to the gout, the rheumatism, and cramp, without making mention of other accidents—what would be the fate of our poor family? Must not the regret of our parents be excessive, at having placed so great a difference between sisters who are so perfectly equal? Alas! we must perish from distress; for it would not be in my power even to scrawl a suppliant petition for relief, having been obliged to employ the hand of another in transcribing the request which I have now the honor to prefer to you.

Condescend, sir, to make my parents sensible of the injustice of an exclusive tenderness, and of the necessity of distributing their care and affection among all their children equally.

> I am, with profound respect, Sirs,
> Your obedient servant,
> THE LEFT HAND

now. After all, regardless of what is going on in students' lives, right this minute they do not have any problems, so they can enjoy being in a quiet room.

If you can shut out worldly concerns and feel momentary relief from pain, this experience gives you a toehold: It proves you can have a good minute—or longer. If you can do it once, you can do it again. Then you can have one good hour, then two. You just keep building.

Students are asked to put all troubles aside and focus on the present. Instead of trying to force any changes, students are led through a yogalike progressive relaxation technique, tensing and relaxing muscles from the tips of their toes to the tops of their heads. They are encouraged to simply listen to their bodies.

The point of this exercise is to learn to relax out in the world. If you chronically let things upset you, it takes a big toll on your body. If you can relax under difficult circumstances, or let go of tension quickly if you become stressed, you are going to be far less vulnerable to negative emotions. Just being aware of how you are feeling, especially where you might be holding tension, is quite useful, because then you can learn to relax those areas. By practicing deep relaxation, you get good at identifying trouble spots. This is a good thing to do while you're standing in line.

At the end of the first session, students receive a tape of the relaxation exercise to practice at home. They also have homework, which is designed to reinforce the workshop material (see box on pages 96–97).

WEEK TWO: BODY TALK

When students return to the Relaxation Workshop the following week, some of them are like different people. Students who were visibly tense the first week are now relaxed and smiling.

In the second session, students learn to "talk" to their bodies in a positive way. Every school-aged child who has gotten a slightly sore throat from sleeping with his mouth open knows he can work that into a full-fledged "cold" if he does not want to go to school that day. Every adult who has not wanted to go to a dinner party knows how to come down with a splitting headache the night of the dreaded event.

Conversely, a teacher of mine who believed in the body/mind connection dryly noted it was interesting how few brides are sick on their wedding day. Indeed, athletes and actors often make astounding recoveries because they do not want to miss a game or a performance.

You can talk yourself into getting better the same way you can talk yourself into getting worse. That is why students are urged to envision themselves how they want to be. You want your body to hear the right message.

The body responds to positive self-talk. This conversation works both ways, like a real conversation where you both speak and listen.

In the second session, students are once again guided through deep relaxation. Then they are encouraged to pose questions to their injuries, such as: Why is the pain there? Is there anything I can do? and (politely, of course) Will all pain please leave now?

This Body Talk technique yields highly specific and valuable information. It is useful to repeat when you feel stuck in recovery.

Four Relaxation Tips

SEND THE RIGHT MESSAGE

Some people will answer the question "How are you feeling?" with one word—"Terrible!" It may be true that they feel awful, but that reply is not such a great message. Your body can hear you, so it responds by feeling worse. If someone asks about *you*, be sure to give the response you want your body to hear. Even "I'm still healing" is a powerfully positive message.

Think of yourself and the other members of the workshop as whole. Here's why: If you focus on your injury, you are in a sense nourishing your disability. Rather, focus on what is right and healthy.

Positive talk works miracles for other people, too. Everyone has enormous power to help everybody else. We can all say to someone, "You're doing great! I'm so glad to see you!" and that person's spirits will lift. Always encourage other RSIers—it is one of the best things you can do for that person.

BE PATIENT WITH THE PACE OF HEALING

If you are impatient, and you keep asking everybody when you are going to get better, you are pushing your body, and it can hear you.

Consider two kinds of bosses. One boss is pushy—somebody

Homework for the Relaxation Workshop

• **Get your physical exercise.** If you don't already have a regular overall exercise program, talk to your doctor or physical therapist about beginning one. Get twenty to forty minutes of vigorous, aerobic exercise three to five times a week in addition to whatever strengthening and stretching exercises you are already doing for RSI. This need not require expensive equipment or great skill; going for a walk fast enough to get your heart rate up is inexpensive and easy.

If you're out of shape, don't overdo it. The goal here is to get yourself in the habit of exercising, so find an activity you like and stick with it. Start slowly and be consistent.

• **Keep a diary.** This does not have to be elaborate. Just record how you are feeling, what improvements you have made—no matter how minute—and any discoveries that have helped you feel better. Do not limit yourself to RSI; write about any aspect of your life. If you cannot write, tape your thoughts. Discontinue the diary if you become obsessive about it.

• **Compose a list of aspirations.** These should cover what you would like to improve about your health and mental outlook. Keep to the present tense, as in *"I am now pain-free, I enjoy doing my exercises, and my optimism grows stronger every day"*—rather than *"I would like to be pain-free and will try to get more exercise and will do my best to keep my spirits up."*

Read your aspirations every day. Embellish the list with better ideas as you go along. Do not let your imagination be bogged down by your own fear or someone else's assessment of your condition: Aim high. See yourself in perfect health. Spend at least fifteen minutes a day visualizing yourself in good health. This is a nice thing to do in the morning.

• **Find a hero.** Choose someone who has overcome tough circumstances in a positive way, and whose story has particular appeal to you. This can be a historic personage or an admired friend or acquaintance. (You can have more than one hero.) Try to emulate this person in your daily life.

• **Think positive.** If you find yourself obsessed with worry, stop for a moment and consciously imagine things easily working out to your benefit. Replace doubt with confidence, worry with serenity, fear with trust, and anger with peace and love.

• **Make up a joke about RSI.** Tell it at the next session. It is best to be original, but if you need help getting started, read a few joke books.

who shouts, "Hurry up, hurry up; what's the matter with you?" You feel tense when that person comes around. Your bile rises as you wait for the crack of the whip.

The other boss never rushes you. This boss makes you feel like a million bucks, and respects you, your work, and your abilities. You can relax and be yourself. For that person, you would gladly make sacrifices.

It is the same way with your body, except this time, you are the boss. Your body wants to heal in its own time, and the pain is telling you in part to stop pushing. So the best thing you can do is be understanding and let it go at its own pace.

TAKE A VACATION FROM RSI

Some RSIers are highly motivated people who approach recovery with the same gusto they had when they were working. Motivation can be great, but so is the occasional day off. Take an RSI vacation day. Do not do anything related to your injury such as calling the doctor or the Workers' Compensation office. Do not commiserate about your injury with friends. Instead, forget about RSI. Go to the movies or immerse yourself in a good book, beautiful music, or works of art.

Just because we are injured does not mean we cannot live fully, enjoy many things about life, and share the warmth of friendship. You do not need money, either. Museums often have free days; public libraries lend audio- and videotapes as well as books.

LAUGH

At her favorite sushi restaurant . . . in San Anselmo, Dyann Dennis noticed the chef wearing a wristband. "Sore," he explained. "Big weekend chopping sashimi."
Dyann: "Whaddya call that, carp and tuna syndrome?"
—ITEM IN HERB CAEN'S COLUMN, *San Francisco Chronicle*

Laughter can ease difficult situations, put things in perspective, and add much pleasure to life, but it is also quite useful as a painkiller. Comedian Buddy Hackett explained the process as follows. There are two kinds of pain: physical and psychological. Laughter is a feeling of release and relief. "When you go *ha ha ha ha*, whatever's hurting you in your head or in your knee, you don't feel either one of those things. And that's the whole story of laughter. Release from pain."

Ellen K. discovered this for herself once while watching a Robin Williams movie on television. "I was laughing so hard I blew up my microwave because I put the potato in for twenty-four minutes instead of twelve," she recalled. It was one of the few times she could recall not feeling pain.

7

THE HEALING POWER OF
EXERCISE AND GOOD POSTURE

Exercise helps you heal in myriad ways. It improves circulation and helps you maintain strength and flexibility. It makes you feel good, so it is great for combating depression. Exercise is one of the best ways to protect yourself against further injuries in other areas of your musculature. Movement stimulates the production of synovial fluid, which lubricates the joints and allows tendons to glide within their sheaths.

The body needs to move in a balanced, moderate fashion to remain healthy. It needs vigorous exercise *and* relaxation, not just a steady diet of rest and immobility. If you don't stretch and strengthen your muscles, they get stiff, sore, and weak.

In the early days of evolution, people got vigorous exercise naturally. Humans had to stay fit: Their lives depended on the strength and agility of their bodies. As hunters—and hunted—our evolutionary ancestors ran and walked for miles. Even as little as one hundred years ago, people got far more exercise during the course of the day than do modern Americans.

As we edge into the twenty-first century, industrialized people use less and less of their total physical capacity at work and more and more of their hands. Many adults never exercise at all. They sit during the commute to work. They sit all day at their desks and then go home at night and sit in front of the television. No wonder so many Americans live in chronic pain.

Sitting for prolonged periods shortens the hamstrings. It slows circulation. It compresses abdominal organs. Blood pools in the feet. As noted earlier, the body frequently starts to take on the dimensions of the chair the person sits on. The spine collapses into a giant C-curve. The chin juts forward, forcing the neck to work hard to support the heavy head. The pectoral muscles contract, and the shoulders slump. The upper back muscles overstretch and can no longer hold the shoulders square.

What you are *not* doing becomes as important as what you are doing. Consider the long-term consequences of static loading. "If you put a joint in immobility for a period of time, you will not be able to move that joint," explained Dr. Cianca. "A classic case is frozen shoulder. A person stops moving their shoulder for some reason, and the joint actually becomes bound down. When they go to move it, it's painful. The synovial fluid works best when the joint is being used. If it gets overused, then you interject other things into the synovial fluid, i.e., inflammatory response and the by-products of that process."

If you do not already have an overall fitness program, do yourself a favor and *start today*. You will gain many benefits, not the least of which will be progress in your recovery.

Beginning Your Exercise Program

When I feel like exercising, I just lie down until the feeling goes away.

—ROBERT M. HUTCHINS, educator

People who have ignored health-preserving advice for years often suddenly snap to attention when they are diagnosed with RSI. When you realize how vital your hands are to every aspect of life, you are in a terrific hurry to get better, so you approach rehabilitation with gusto.

Enthusiasm is terrific, but before you plunge into vigorous exercise, learn the proper approach.

GET PROFESSIONAL GUIDANCE

When you learn a new exercise, it should be done under the careful supervision of a physical or occupational therapist. Exercising in improper alignment could exacerbate your problem or create new ones.

People have differing needs in terms of supervision. A person with a lot of athletic or dance training may need little attention. Beginners may feel they need someone to watch every repetition until they have mastered a movement.

YOU NEED A PERSONAL PLAN

Every injury is unique; therefore, no single exercise plan will be appropriate for every person. Be cautious about following an exercise program you see in a magazine or newspaper. Some exercises would be harmful to someone in the acute stages of RSI. While a movement might be safe in most cases, it could be dangerous for people with certain injuries—and you need to know which exercises are right for you.

The other problem with doing exercises from pictures is that you risk performing them the wrong way.

THE EXERCISE TRIAD

A well-rounded exercise program contains three components: strength training, flexibility, and aerobic conditioning. Strength training develops muscles, flexibility keeps them long, and aerobic activity keeps your heart healthy.

Flexibility training is especially critical as we age. In a study of older people, those who participated in a stretch class reported feeling less pain in their daily lives, while those who focused on endurance and strength noted somewhat more pain than before, noted Abby King, assistant professor of health research and policy and medicine at Stanford University School of Medicine.

Do not neglect stretching. To stretch safely, hold the stretch *under* the point of pain and keep breathing. Do not bounce.

CHOOSING AN EXERCISE PROGRAM

It is important to select an exercise program you like. If you are not having fun, you will be less likely to exercise consistently. People who love the great outdoors might consider running on a treadmill a bore; but that may be the perfect solution for someone who likes the idea of exercising in her own home, listening to her favorite music.

GET A TOTAL-BODY WORKOUT

While it is important to gain upper-body strength and flexibility, do not limit your exercise program to that area alone. Keeping your leg, buttocks, and abdominal muscles strong, for instance, will help because you will not need to rely as much on your arms to help you rise from a seated position. You will also be able to get out of bed more easily in the morning if these areas are strong.

The exercises you choose should strengthen the muscles that assist good posture and those that stabilize the shoulder blade (the rhomboids, mid-trapezius, and serratus anterior, which are located on your mid-back).

Be sure to stretch the chest and neck muscles (pectorals, scalenes, and upper trapezius) and the muscles that bend and straighten the wrist.

TIMING COUNTS

Doing your exercises first thing in the morning makes sense for two important reasons. First, you are less likely to skip your routine if you do it right away. Second, exercise stimulates synovial fluid, which lubricates the joints and tendon sheaths of the body. This prepares the body for work and helps prevent injury.

HOW TO DO YOUR EXERCISES

Work the major muscle first so you don't fatigue smaller muscles.

When in doubt, do less. Use lighter weights and perform fewer repetitions, rather than letting eagerness to heal lead to injury.

Always maintain proper alignment. Hold your abdomen in. Keep your neck and shoulders relaxed. If you have trouble maintaining good form, ask for a simpler exercise.

Work through the entire range of motion to develop even muscle strength.

Keep breathing from the diaphragm.

STICKING WITH YOUR PROGRAM

When it comes to why they do not exercise, people will come up with a variety of excuses. But, with apologies to Irving Berlin, there is no discipline like self-discipline.

What if you're too busy to exercise? Make time for it. If you really can't fit your whole routine in, do an abbreviated version, at least a few quick stretches, a few strengthening exercises.

What should you do if you don't feel like exercising one day? Do it anyway. You'll usually feel better afterward.

EXERCISING IN GROUPS OR PAIRS

Exercise groups are great because they give you energy and motivation. If you have an inspiring aerobics instructor, for instance, she will also keep things fresh, interesting, and challenging. Many people enjoy the social aspect of exercise as much as the physical benefits.

You will be more likely to stick with your routine if someone will notice that you have not been around. Be sure your instructor understands your limitations. If you think an activity is dangerous for you, trust your own feelings and discontinue it.

Some people find it hard to stay on exercise programs. But if you get into the habit, you will one day be genuinely disappointed if something interferes with your routine.

SOLO EXERCISE

Disciplined RSIers can choose activities they can do on their own, like swimming, running, or doing aerobics with videotapes.

You can also hire a personal trainer, but make sure that person understands that you have special needs. It is a good idea to have your trainer call your physician or physical therapist to discuss your program.

REVISE YOUR EXERCISE PLAN PERIODICALLY

You might need to adjust your exercise program frequently for many reasons. As your symptoms ebb and flow, you might be able to do certain exercises when you are feeling strong, but they might be too much a week later.

Sometimes people relapse, so a lighter routine may be indicated. And when your program feels too easy, you might need to add resistance by using heavier weights or a stronger elastic band

---

Workout Tips

- Exercise done mindlessly is not as effective as that performed with good concentration.
- Do not resent exercising—you're just working against yourself if you do. The more fun you can have, the better.
- When you exercise, see yourself getting stronger and more flexible with each repetition.
- Exercise opportunistically. If you have only five or ten minutes, use that time. It is better than not moving at all. March in place during television commercials or extended telephone conversations. Take the stairs instead of the elevator. Walk instead of drive.

TRAVEL TIPS

- Take elastic bands, which are lightweight, for resistance.
- When you are a houseguest, substitute soup cans for dumbbells.
- If you are staying in a hotel with a pool, use children's inflatable water wings for resistance in the water (wear them on your biceps or ankles).

---

to get the most benefit. This way, you can continue building strength until you reach your maintenance level.

Cautions About Exercise

THE RIGHT AMOUNT OF EXERCISE

Any exercise can be harmful if overdone, so pay attention to how you are feeling. When you find your maintenance level, stop adding weights and repetitions, because that can lead to overuse injuries.

Healthy people will be able to exercise differently from those doing rehabilitation exercise. For instance, an uninjured person might be able to lift light weights right away, whereas a person with RSI will add weights only gradually, under the supervision of a rehabilitation therapist. Exercise machines cannot always be adjusted for big or small people, so they may not be appropriate for you if your body cannot be properly aligned while performing a movement. You may also have to avoid machines with handheld grips.

You are at risk of overtraining if you get inadequate rest, use improper technique, train too hard on consecutive days, increase activities too quickly, or do not cut back after brief lapses in your program. Soreness is considered a muscle injury—take it seriously!

Signs of overtraining include chronic muscle or joint soreness, remaining fatigued well after your workout, irritability, lack of interest in training, declining performance, and increased incidence of colds and infections. Avoid overtraining—it can lead to overuse injuries!

EXERCISING WITH A DISABILITY

In some cases, it may be hard to find an exercise program that does not aggravate your symptoms. For instance, it may be too painful to run if you have RSI because the bouncing hurts your arms.

Do not allow this to deter you. Even severely disabled people can benefit from exercise. Speak to your physician or a trainer with expertise in designing programs for people with disabilities. An injury in one part of your body is no reason to let the rest of yourself go.

My Daily Workout

I always have gotten lots of exercise, but, like many women, I did not focus on strengthening the muscles of my upper body. After my injury, I began weight training to develop strength. I started by training my upper body but eventually added exercises for all the major muscle groups, to ensure no muscle group was neglected.

Most days, I spend about thirty to forty-five minutes working out with light weights. Endurance—not power lifting—is my goal, so I do thirty repetitions of each exercise.

For strength, flexibility, good posture, and aerobic training, I study ballet four times a week. Each class lasts an hour and a half, not counting stretch time. I walk to physical therapy appointments and ballet classes as often as possible, which takes an hour round trip. At night, I usually do another round of stretching before I go to sleep. When I'm in the country, I love to hike.

On those rare occasions when I do not have time for my full routine, I content myself with an abbreviated workout; but I always do *something*—either a walk, or ballet, or my resistance routine—and I always make a point of stretching frequently.

While my routine seems like too much to some people, I need a lot of exercise, and have found that this routine is right for me, just as you and your physical therapist will find the right balance for you. And even though I am doing very well in recovery, I still have to work at it every day.

RSI-Friendly Exercises

WALKING AND HIKING

Walking is one of the best things you can do. If done at a brisk pace, walking can raise your heart rate, infuse the lungs with oxygen, and gently stretch and strengthen your muscles.

In his book *Spontaneous Healing,* Dr. Andrew Weil explains another benefit of walking. "When you walk, the movement of your limbs is cross-patterned: the right leg and the left arm move forward at the same time, then the left leg and right arm. This type of movement generates electrical activity in the brain that has a harmonizing effect on the whole central nervous system—a special benefit of walking that you do not necessarily get from other kinds of exercise."

Hiking in steep mountainous locales is a great cardiovascular exercise, especially going uphill. Be cautious about heavy backpacks, particularly if you have thoracic outlet syndrome or other neck problems. Ask your doctor or rehabilitation therapist for advice.

SWIMMING AND POOL AEROBICS

If you avoid strokes that aggravate symptoms, swimming can be beneficial for people with RSI. One woman supported her chest with a Styrofoam paddleboard to reduce strain on her arms.

Pool aerobics can be a terrific cardiovascular workout. There are many advantages to working in water: Your weight is suspended, so the risk of knee, foot, and ankle injuries is reduced. You can use the water as resistance. If you are overweight or self-conscious about moving, the water protects you somewhat from feeling scrutinized.

YOGA

Yoga can help people maintain flexibility and breathe better, and it can be very relaxing and invigorating. Be careful to avoid the movements that stress your hands and neck, such as the Downward Dog, Frog, Plow, or Shoulder Stand.

Activities to Avoid

Hand-intensive activities such as tennis, volleyball, bowling, racquetball, skiing, boxing, karate, biking, and power lifting are not advisable.

It is also best to avoid push-ups, chin-ups, rings, and any exercise machine that requires a hand grip. If you enjoy working out on cross-country skiing or rowing machines, ask an occupational therapist how to rig a harness to attach to your upper arm—so that you can get the benefit without the hand strain.

Do not use handheld or ankle weights during aerobics classes; it is too difficult to control the movement and could lead to injury.

Do not squeeze rubber balls, use hand exercisers, or do wrist curls unless you have a competent physician's approval and are carefully supervised by a rehabilitation therapist!

The Therapeutic Power of Proper Posture

Posture and exercise go together, because strong, flexible muscles hold your bones in place. Movement should be performed in proper alignment or it can be dangerous.

Toddlers naturally have perfect posture. Their heads sit poised atop their spines; their backs are straight. It is a joy to behold. If they could only maintain good alignment when they grow up!

If you look at old photographs, you often see adults, even those of advanced age, who still hold themselves erect, probably as a result of parental admonitions to stand up straight. Today good posture is more the exception than the rule.

The importance of learning good posture in childhood and maintaining it throughout life cannot be overstated. When the bones are well aligned, with knees, hips, shoulders, and head balanced over the feet, the muscles can maintain their proper length, allowing them to work efficiently and without strain.

AVOID THE HEAD-FORWARD POSITION

The human head weighs approximately ten pounds. When it is carried three inches forward from the body's center of gravity, it adds an extra thirty pounds to the neck, as Rene Cailliet, M.D., pointed out.

The head-forward position can compress nerves that nourish the hand and arm. It also compresses blood vessels, choking off the supply to the hand and arm. The muscles of the neck and upper back become overstretched and weakened.

"Forward head, rounded shoulders, tight anterior muscles, weak posterior muscles, all crowd the neurovascular structure as it passes through the thoracic outlet," explained Dr. Cianca. "Poor posture sets up somebody for injury farther down the upper extremity. The farther out the structure, the more dependent it is on the structures above it."

In most offices, the majority of people sit with craned necks staring at computer screens. This posture is also extremely common during another ubiquitous daily activity—reading. Years ago, schoolchildren were taught to sit with their feet flat on the floor, the book held at a forty-five-degree angle resting on the table. I cannot remember the last time I saw someone use this position. Most of the time, the reading material lies flat on the table, with the reader's head and shoulder slumped over it. Sometimes you will see readers lounge in their chairs, feet atop the desk, spines curved.

STAND TALL REGARDLESS OF HEIGHT

To stand properly, the weight should balance between two feet. The head should align with the ears over the shoulders, which are in line with the pelvis. The abdominal muscles should be held in without interfering with breathing. The chin should be level, not looking up or down. Think of Audrey Hepburn as she enters the ball in *My Fair Lady*, with her long neck and perfectly level chin.

To feel a "straight" spine (though technically the spine has natural curves in good posture), it is sometimes easier for beginners to feel the spine elongate while lying on the floor than standing.

Many images are used to suggest the proper standing position. Some people imagine they are suspended like a marionette by a cord going out the top of their head. Others think of the head floating like a balloon, spine dropping easily beneath it. Or you can think of pushing toward the sky from the top of the head.

SIT UP

Working at computers with poor posture makes people sitting ducks for injury. If you are forced by circumstances to sit in a chair that does not support your spine, sit on the edge of the seat and use your muscles to sit tall instead of slouching against the backrest.

If you must lean forward while seated, do so by bending from the hip joint, keeping the head, chest, and pelvis in a straight line, as though your spine were inflexible. Slouching crowds the lungs.

MAINTAINING GOOD POSTURE WHILE CARRYING THINGS

When I look at pictures of people in other countries walking with baskets atop their heads, I am struck by their posture. This mode of carrying burdens makes good sense, leaving the hands free and the shoulders unstressed.

We carry shoulder bags and briefcases, which distribute burdens lopsidedly. Over the years, this habit often results in marked elevation of one shoulder and depression of the other. People who use heavy backpacks frequently round their shoulders forward and crane their necks.

The Equestrian Trick

A riding enthusiast shared this trick, which equestrians use to maintain proper posture: Lift your arms above your head and stretch your hands to the sky. You will feel your rib cage lift and your spine elongate. Now bring your arms to a relaxed position by your sides, shoulders down, but keep your rib cage suspended above your waist just as when you were reaching overhead.

The Book Trick

Years ago, finishing schools taught girls to walk with books balanced on their heads to encourage good posture. This is a great way to sense true verticality, because if your chin is too high or low, the book will fall off. Use a fairly heavy clothbound book, such as a dictionary, so it won't slip off your hair too easily.

First, stand with the book on your head. Slowly turn your head from right to left without letting the book slide. Next, walk around the house with the book balanced on your head. Finally, sit with the book on your head. This is how straight you should be all the time, which means you will not be resting your spine against the backrest, but rather using your own muscles to hold yourself erect.

WATCH YOURSELF IN THE MIRROR

Besides being one of the best retraining tools, mirrors are plentiful and inexpensive. Study your posture often. If you catch your reflection in a store window, notice whether you are slouching.

Some people get tremendously self-conscious when they stand tall. They fear people will think they are conceited. This is not the case at all. In fact, people who have good posture radiate good health, self-confidence, and poise. That makes you more approachable, not less.

Good posture needs to be practiced until it becomes automatic, and bad posture feels wrong.

8

PROTECTING YOUR HANDS DURING DAILY ACTIVITIES

People knock their knuckles against hard surfaces, yell at their hands, and grasp objects in a death grip even when it hurts to do so. This is no way to treat the part of the anatomy that anthropologists credit with the evolution of humankind. The hand—particularly the opposable thumb—separates us from other primates, and it took millennia of patient use to allow us to evolve into the cerebral beings that we are. What other tool is versatile enough to repair a watch, sense warmth and cold, cradle a child, *and* break a brick? Yet people treat their computer systems with far more respect—after all, they may have cost thousands of dollars!

No amount of money, and no doctor on Earth, can restore the full use of your hands if you damage them beyond repair.

General Hand-Saving Principles

Living with RSI teaches you to spare your hands during all daily activities. Though most RSIers learn this quickly, it surprised me that so many people did not protect their hands as well as they could. This was the stimulus for a workshop I developed, called Tricks and Tips for People with RSI. As might be expected, some of the best ideas came from RSIers themselves.

Obviously, your injury may prevent you from taking advantage of every tip presented here. Use only those that help.

TUNE IN TO YOUR BODY

Most RSIers experienced warning signs of injury months and sometimes years before they finally saw a doctor. Learn to listen to your body. Get into the habit of tuning in to your body frequently during the day. Catching injury when it is just beginning is the best way to prevent it from becoming chronic.

Paying attention is particularly crucial if you are using different parts of your body in new ways. If you alternate hands, notice how you tend to grip too tightly with the nondominant hand and correct that tendency before it has a chance to become habitual or develop into a substitution injury.

BEWARE OF REPETITIVE MOVEMENTS

In their attempt to make good use of downtime, people often do other repetitive tasks during breaks. "I didn't understand that *any* repetitive motion would hurt my hands," explained Lynette C., who had a flare-up from doing a lot of filing when she could not use her keyboard.

You don't have to be totally idle when you are resting from work, but avoid repetitive or strenuous movements.

AVOID UNNECESSARY COMPUTING

One man associated the onset of his injury with an upsurge in computer use because of the hours he was spending on the Internet. Now he phones people rather than answering e-mail by computer. Think about your priorities, and save your hands for essential tasks.

BE KIND TO YOUR HANDS

Once, after a workshop, one of my students repeatedly slapped her hands against her thighs in frustration at her inability to use them. Her emotions were perfectly understandable, but I finally said, "Please don't. You must be kind to your hands. They can't get well if you keep hitting them." She immediately seemed to understand that she was sending the wrong message to her body. It is hard to heal if you keep beating up your hands.

BE OBSERVANT

Take advantage of your powers of observation before you use force. Watch someone else open a door before you struggle with it, only to find it is locked. Notice whether the sign says "Push" or "Pull" and which side of the door the handle is on.

Think about your own flare-up triggers and analyze how they happen.

JOIN FORCES

Leaving the building after a Tricks and Tips Workshop, several RSIers clustered at a revolving door. One went ahead, pushing the door with her hand. If two of them had pushed, preferably using their shouders, neither would have experienced as much strain. Look for opportunities to use combined strength, especially with other RSIers.

USE HAND-SAVING TOOLS WHENEVER POSSIBLE

Instead of straining your hands, use pliers, scissors, and wrenches to help you. Keep tools handy anywhere you use them: the office, kitchen, and bathroom.

Tools may have duel uses. One woman used a salad fork to press the buttons of a microwave. Bottle can openers can break the vacuum of artichoke jar lids. Foam hair curlers can be slipped over pencils and forks to make them easier to hold.

ROLL, SLIDE, OR WHEEL

When moving a heavy object, slide it; do not lift it. Use rolling wastebaskets and laundry carts.

USE POWER MUSCLES

Whenever possible, use the big muscles of your back and torso rather than the fine muscles of your hands to perform a task.

The Hand Bank

Most of the time, when your injury has stabilized, you realize you have limited use of your hands. Think of the amount of hand energy you have during the day as the daily allowance in your "Hand Bank."

Here are some hints on budgeting well:

• **Do less.** Doing less than you want to on a given day is hard, but it is the only way to keep flare-ups at bay. Refraining from certain activities entirely is especially difficult with deeply ingrained cultural rituals, such as shaking hands and holding doors open for other people.

• **Think first.** When faced with an activity you know causes flare-ups, ask yourself if there is another approach to the task that will not stress your hands.

• **Prioritize.** One woman said she prioritized her activities by asking if it was worth being in pain for a week. If it is more important to cuddle the cat than to clean the living room, ignore the dust balls.

• **Plan ahead.** When you understand your symptoms, you can plan around them. "I learned to cut my grapefruit at night before I go to sleep, because my hands are too stiff to do it in the morning," one woman reported.

Choosing the Right Tools

A well-balanced tool designed to fit the hand and the movement it requires is a joy to use. Conversely, a tool that requires contorting one's body around its design makes work miserable. If only we could convince tool designers to consider the hapless soul who will be forced to use their creations day in and day out!

Here are some pointers about choosing tools:

- Tools should come in several sizes.
- Whenever possible, choose a tool that fits your hand. The tool—not the wrist—should bend.
- Avoid grooved handles. As one wit at the New Zealand Department of Labor observed, "Grooves usually fit only the hand of the designer!" A textured grip covering is better.
- Metal handles are cold and slippery. Choose soft covering to cushion hands from sharp edges, allow a more relaxed grip, and protect hands from heat and cold.

DON'T BE A DO-IT-YOURSELFER

Heavy activities such as painting, construction, and gardening are better left to those who are not injured.

The Specifics of Everyday Life

PREPARING AND EATING MEALS

A proper diet is important for healing; preparing your own meals helps you ensure good nutrition. Because of their injuries, shop-

- Triggers should use at least two—and up to four—fingers. The middle part of the finger should be used to pull it.
- Electric tools save repetitive hand movements.
- Avoid tools that vibrate.
- Avoid handles that cut into the palm.
- Left-handed people should select tools designed for the left hand, or tools that can be used by either right- or left-handed people.
- Some tools can be used with two hands together, which reduces the strain on the dominant hand.
- When tools open and close, spring-loaded action is helpful.
- Tools should not be so large that they are hard to put your hands around nor so small that they are difficult to hold.
- Heavy tools should be well balanced.

Tools, gadgets, and gizmos can be expensive. If possible, try them out before you buy. Patronize merchants who have a generous return policy, or borrow a product from a friend before you purchase one of your own.

---

ping, cooking, and even eating are difficult for many RSIers, though. Here are some tips to help you with the troublesome aspects.

Grocery Shopping
- Do not buy the large size of any product unless someone can help you lift it.
- Transfer heavy items like dish-washing liquid and laundry detergent to smaller vessels for daily use.
- Buy prechopped garlic and precut vegetables. Hint: Frozen peas or corn can double as ice packs.
- When you are shopping, lock heavy valuables such as gym

bags or briefcases in the trunk of your car instead of carrying them around with you.
- Have your groceries delivered.
- Tell the bagger to put your purchases in several small, light bags rather than one big sack.
- Ask the clerks or other shoppers to lift things from the shelf for you.

Cooking Tips
- Scissors are indispensable in the kitchen. They can be used to trim fat from meat, open stubborn packaging, and snip string beans.
- Kitchenware stores carry a wide variety of soft-handled tools, such as pizza cutters, graters, and steak knives designed for people with fragile hands.
- There are special devices to open jars and bottles; check hardware stores or the catalogs in the resource guide.
- Pots that have two generous handles on either side will be easier to hold than those with a single or short handle.
- If it hurts you to use twist ties, close bags with a clothespin.
- When you are buying cooking utensils and baking pans, choose brands with easy-to-clean coating.
- Ziploc bags with zippers are easier to use than ones you must press shut, but catalogs also sell a tool to help you close Ziploc bags.
- Be sure to have an assortment of good knives. Make sure each knife is well balanced and that the handle fits comfortably in your hand. Serrated knives will make it easier to slice tomatoes and bread.
- Use lightweight housewares. Cast-iron skillets are a great source of iron, but they are heavy, and thus tough for RSIers to use. Get lightweight cooking pans instead. The same goes for those gorgeous but heavy earthenware plates and serving dishes. Save them for days when someone else is helping with dinner.
- Many RSIers use paper or plastic dinnerware. Paper plates can be reinforced with woven holders.
- Plastic is lighter than glass, especially when filled with liquid, so use plastic measuring cups, pitchers, and tumblers.

- Catalogs carry cutting boards with nails to skewer vegetables so you can slice them with one hand. When cutting, angle the food, not your wrist.
- If you tend to drop things a lot, do potentially messy jobs over the sink so accidents will be easier to clean up. Also, put a plastic-covered rack on the bottom of the sink to avoid breakage.

Eating

- One man suggests eating Thai style to avoid the pain of having to spear food with your fork: Push the food (which will be cut into bite-sized pieces) onto the fork with a spoon.
- When dining out, if you are ordering food that is not usually prepared in bite-sized pieces, you may also ask that the food be cut in the kitchen before it is served.
- Substitute difficult-to-cut foods with easier ones; for instance, instead of a steak, have a tender piece of salmon.
- If bringing the utensil to your mouth aggravates an elbow injury, it may be less painful to let the movement come from the shoulder. You also might train your nondominant hand for eating, but be sure to stay relaxed.

SLEEPING

Sleeping well helps the entire body heal, but many RSIers lie awake from neck or wrist pain. One woman could find relief only by sleeping on a hardwood floor. Another used "a million pillows, rearranged" under her arms to elevate them.

Gadgets like cervical pillows go only so far. Sometimes neck pain is solved not by a special pillow, but by physical therapy. (See the discussion of biofeedback in chapter 6.)

If you dislike sleeping in the rigid splints your physician has prescribed, here is one way to keep your elbows straight while you sleep: Fold a thick bath towel in half, wrap it around your elbow (not too tightly), and pin it closed. This will prevent you from flexing your elbow in your sleep. You can also do this for your wrists using a facecloth.

Some RSIers find it very difficult to sleep with splints on. Try soft splints or gloves. Be sure to talk to your doctor before using *any* splint.

OPENING DOORS

Most doors seem to be built for fullbacks or power lifters, certainly not for bantamweight women with modest upper-body strength. Some doors conspire to confound you—they perversely want to be pulled when you thought they wanted to be pushed. They slam shut before you have fully exited or entered. Door handles do not always operate as expected, either. You think a doorknob will be perfectly straightforward, but no—this one turns *counterclockwise*.

You never realize how many doors you open every day until you develop RSI. Here are some tips for negotiating an entrance or exit when there's no one around to help you:

- Pushing doors open is relatively easy, because you can use your hips or shoulder. But heavy doors that pull inward are troublesome. Instead of pulling a door open with your arm outstretched, stand close to it, turn the handle, and walk backward, holding your arm still so you can use as much of your leg and back strength as possible.
- With revolving doors, take advantage of natural laws. A revolving door will require less pressure to move if you push on its outer edge rather than toward the center. Let someone else go first to get the momentum going.
- Some buses have strips that assist opening. Use them. Notice whether someone else has rung for your stop so you do not ring unnecessarily.
- If a doorbell is out of order, and the mere thought of knocking on a door sets off an episode of pain, do not rap with your knuckles. Tap with an umbrella or other object, or kick the door with your feet. Better yet, call from a pay phone and tell someone to wait for you at the door.
- To push elevator buttons, use your elbow or knuckles to reduce forearm strain.

READING

Once people become injured, they start noticing their posture in all kinds of settings. As with computing, the most comfortable reading position over the long run is proper seated posture. Bring the book to you; do not crane your neck to read.

The following items will help make reading a more comfortable activity for you:

- **The reading chair.**   Most people read in any old chair, but do yourself a favor and purchase a reading chair with good back support and padded arms.

- **Reading stands.**   Propping books on reading stands allows you to keep your neck straight while you read. If reading at a table or desk, use a reading stand or build a platform with other books.

- **Reading pillows.**   You may not have to hold your book if you pile pillows on your lap while reading. Use enough pillows so that you do not have to bend your neck to see the page. Rough fabrics (such as corduroy or tweed) and soft pillows (filled with kapok, beans, and down) are easier to manipulate than hard pillows covered with slippery fabrics. Ready-made reading pillows with sewn-in book holders and bookmarks can be purchased by catalog.

- **Hardbound books.**   Some RSIers find that hard- or spiral-bound books are easier to hold than paperbacks.

- **Weighted bookmarks.**   Leather bookmarks with lead weights on each end make it unnecessary for you to hold open the book.

- **Page-turning devices.**   Many RSIers find it painful to turn pages of books and magazines. A pencil can serve as a simple page-turning device: Use the eraser end to help lift the page, then carefully slide your hand beneath it and turn it as though flipping a pancake. Or order one of the turning devices available through catalogs (see resources).

WATCHING TV

One of my clients realized that when she watched television, she craned her neck. She usually sat on the couch, which was too soft to support good posture.

Get a good reading chair, or support your spine in proper alignment with pillows.

SHAKING HANDS

The handshake is an important social lubricant, but it can be excruciating to some RSIers. Shaking hands poses the following dilemma:
Although you want to be polite, people are often introduced fleet-
ingly, and you may not wish to divulge your condition to every person you meet.

RSIers tend to be very inventive about this. Some people refuse
to shake altogether; some withdraw their hands slightly when they
shake, so if the other person has a bone-crushing grip, only their
fingertips will feel the pressure. One woman keeps her fingers
slightly curved to avoid overenthusiastic squeezes; another offers
her elbow.

Once, when a severely injured man, Herbert H., talked with me
after a presentation, a colleague joined us, hand extended. It would
be very painful for Herbert to shake, so I quickly said, "You don't
have to shake hands!"

The other man, without missing a beat, said, "We'll bow," and
gallantly bent at the waist.

One RSIer said in her circle everyone slapped hands in a high
five to greet one another. "I guess I'm going to have to change my
friends," she said wryly. Of course, real friends will make accommodations to avoid causing you pain.

If shaking hands is painful for you, find a way to refuse that is
gracious to the other person and comfortable for you. Do not stress
your hands just to be sociable.

If you suspect someone might have RSI, always ask if he or she
wants to shake before offering your hand.

WRITING

Some RSIers find handwriting far more comfortable than using a
computer; for others, even signing a check is agony. If writing is
painful for you, avoid it whenever you can. Use address labels. Ask
other people to help you fill in forms.

Creative Hand-Saving

THE FLOWER TRICK

Linda J. Johnson, a California occupational therapist, once helped a panic-stricken mother-of-the-bride who dreaded shaking hands in the receiving line. "I told her to hold her bouquet with both hands and nod her head," Linda said with a chuckle.

If you do not have flowers handy, use a coffee mug, book, or purse. Former Senate Majority Leader Bob Dole does not have RSI, but he suffered a severe arm wound during the Second World War. He always carries a pen in his injured hand (so people will not be tempted to shake it), offering his other hand instead.

THE E.T. HANDSHAKE

When greeting friends with RSI, I sometimes softly touch my forefinger to theirs, as in the *Creation of Adam* by Michelangelo in the Sistine Chapel or the poster for the film *E.T.*

APPLAUDING

Clapping is another one of those social niceties that people with normal hands do as a matter of course, but RSIers dread.

If clapping hurts your hands, substitute any of the following: whistle, shout "Brava" or "Bravo," stamp your feet, gently put your hands together in a nonpercussive fashion (miming the action instead of doing it), or lightly tap your program into your palm.

One way to write less is to develop your memory instead of writing so many notes. Today, people rely on all manner of memory aids, from electronic notebooks to grocery and "to do" lists. But before the invention of the printing press, books were scarce, so they relied on mnemonic systems "to provide storage spaces for the myriad concepts that make up the sum of our human knowledge," as Jonathan Spence noted in *Memory Palace of Matteo Ricci*. As incredible as it seems, friends of Ricci, a sixteenth-century Italian missionary, claimed he could recite volumes of Chinese classics after scanning them once.

Before you automatically start taking notes, think about training your memory. It is not as hard as you think, if you concentrate. During my Tricks and Tips Workshops, students are encouraged to pay attention instead of taking notes. Later, they will use this trick when the need arises, as in opening doors.

If you must write:

- Do not press through forms. Photocopy them instead.
- Do not grip the pen tightly.
- Use a pen that flows freely without pressure. Some RSIers find that wide-barreled fountain pens require little pressure to use. One woman likes to use a soft lead drawing pencil she found at an art supply store.
- Pen expanders—available at stationers and through catalogs—can be very useful because they widen the barrel, which helps some people relax their grip. Three-sided expanders do not roll away when you drop them. Foam hair curlers also work great—some RSIers like to wrap them with electrician's tape.
- Students should consider buying a tape recorder that is powerful enough to pick up the lecturer's voice if they sit at the back of the room. Before purchasing any recorder, be sure the control buttons are easy to operate.

Household Tips

The notion of being envious of someone else's ability to do housework might seem odd to uninjured people. But if you have only limited use of your hands, the idea of giving your house a thorough cleaning—and feeling the joy of immaculate surroundings—might be enough to make you salivate.

The following tips may make household chores less stressful for you.

• **Lower your standards.** Ignoring dust balls and dirty dishes can be difficult for neat freaks, but getting upset about things you cannot change will only raise your stress level.

• **Look for shortcuts.** For example, if you put a wet paper towel over powdered cleanser, the stain will disappear like magic. Just powder the spot, dampen the towel, and walk away for a while.

• **Use a cleaning service.** If you can afford it, hire household help for the heavy stuff, like changing the linen and scrubbing the floor. Consider bartering; find something you can do for willing friends.

• **Do small loads of laundry.** Do not save it up. It will be less stressful to do small, frequent loads. Consider using a laundry service for heavy items like sheets and towels; it may not cost you much more than doing it yourself.

• **Steam instead of iron.** Some garments will lose their wrinkles if you hang them in a steamy bathroom for a while. This trick saves you both time and energy.

• **Learn a new way of vacuuming.** Keep the handle close to you, as though the vacuum were Ginger Rogers and you were Fred Astaire. Then move the handle with your whole body instead of pushing it with your arm.

If you're buying a vacuum, a lightweight model with a wand will be less difficult to use than a heavy upright. Some people can't vacuum because of the vibration of the machine. If you fall into that category, you might consider purchasing a carpet sweeper and covering the handle with dense foam.

CHILDPROOF CAPS

New child-resistant caps will be in place in January 1998 that will be easier for older people to use as well as protect against child poisoning. This will also help some pharmacists who were developing RSI from repeatedly opening and closing childproof containers.

Look for over-the-counter drugs in non-child-resistant containers, which will be labeled as such. For prescription drugs, ask your pharmacist to give you an easy-to-open cap (and keep it out of children's reach). Assistive openers are also available through catalogs.

BATHROOM REMODELING

If you are remodeling your bathroom or kitchen, install hand-friendly faucets, drawer handles, and other hardware. You never realize how many times you turn on a light switch unless it hurts your hands to do so.

One woman with severe trigger finger found it much easier to use faucets with one long handle because she could push it up with the top of her hand and position it to the hot or cold setting by keeping her hand in the handshake position rather than having to twist knobs.

Install counters at a comfortable chopping height. Linoleum floors can be swept if you have trouble vacuuming. Choose flat nap rather than deep-pile carpeting.

Personal Care

SOAP DISPENSERS

Like doors, most soap dispensers are masterpieces of deplorable design. How many times have you wasted hand energy trying to get soap from what turns out to be an empty container? Carry packets of disposable towelettes, soapless hand cleanser, or use bar soap if it's available.

Do not use your fingers to push down the handle of liquid hand soap containers. Instead, make a loose fist and press the spout in the handshake position. This enables you to use bigger muscles instead of straining your hands.

Rather than squeezing shampoo out of the bottle, unscrew the cap and pour it on. Store half-used bottles upside down so you do not have to shake or squeeze them.

BRUSHING TEETH

Electric toothbrushes are useful if the upward and downward motion of brushing hurts. Some people like angled toothbrushes, because they do not have to twist their hands as much to use them.

EASY-TO-WEAR CLOTHING

Avoid shoes with difficult laces and shirts with troublesome buttons or back zippers, unless you have someone to help you dress.

Not only do shoehorns save your hands, they also protect your shoes. Use the long-handled variety to avoid back strain.

PANTY HOSE

There are devices to help you put on panty hose and socks. Avoid control-top nylons; they require a lot of strength to pull on.

PURSES, TOTE BAGS, AND BRIEFCASES

Clean out your bag! Is it really necessary to drag half your earthly possessions everywhere you go? Avoid shoulder bags entirely; belt bags are better. Avoid backpacks unless they place the weight on your hips.

The next time you are looking for a parka, vest, or jacket, choose one with oversized pockets. Big pockets are handy for carrying your keys, wallet—even magazines or paperback books.

The Telephone

HEADSETS

Telephone headsets are not luxuries if your hands fatigue or fall asleep when you hold up a receiver. In addition, headsets ensure that you do not strain your neck by cradling the phone while you use your hands for something else. Most people cradle the phone far more than they think, especially while looking up a number in the phone book or writing something down when they are talking to someone.

Cordless models are especially convenient, because in addition to freeing your hands for other tasks—such as cooking, writing, or looking for something in a folder—you are not tethered to one area. (For more information about headsets, see page 153.)

THE KEYPAD

It's amazing how hard the action is on most Touch-Tone phones. Look for phones that have an easy touch in electronics stores and catalogs.

AUTOMATIC DIALERS

Using the telephone touchpad can be painful. Take advantage of automatic or voice-activated dialing devices; check with your telephone company or look in catalogs (see Resources).

SPECIAL SERVICES FOR PEOPLE WITH DISABILITIES

Some telephone companies offer helpful equipment and services to people with disabilities, including RSI. They will sell you adaptive equipment such as headsets at wholesale cost; or, in some states, you receive it free if your annual salary is less than a certain figure.

You might also receive free services such as directory or operator assistance with dialing numbers. Call your local telephone company and ask what is available. Your physician will probably need to certify that you need the equipment.

The Home Office

Here are seven tips to make things easier for you when you work in your home office:

• **Filing.** When lifting a file folder out of the drawer, put your fingers underneath the entire folder instead of pulling from the tab end. Of course, for this trick to work, you need to get your whole fist into the drawer—which means you cannot overstuff filing cabinets!

• **Opening packages.** Ripping open a supersticky envelope requires a lot of effort. So does opening cardboard boxes that are stapled shut. Do not use your bare hands; use scissors or a razor-style opener for mail and a mat knife for boxes.

• **Electric staplers.** Stapling can be hard on your hands—buy an electric stapler. Many copy machines have these built in.

• **Staple removers.** Look for staple removers that resemble letter openers; they are much easier on your hands.

• **Hole punches.** Put the three-hole punch on the floor and use your feet to operate it. (This works for staplers, too, in a pinch.)

• **Bulletin boards.** Use T-pins to fasten notices to the bulletin board instead of thumbtacks or pushpins, because their shape allows you to pull them out more easily.

• **Folding papers.** If you have to fold papers, do not press hard to make creases. Fold them lightly, then sit on a stack. You'll get a flat crease without the strain. You can also crease papers by piling heavy books on them. (Don't lift a stack of books all at once; do it one at a time.)

On the Road with RSI

CARS

Car seats present many of the same problems that chairs do: People come in all shapes and sizes, but car seats do not. Ideally, car seats should allow you to sit upright and reach foot pedals and gearshifts without strain. Some RSIers have special car seats installed if they like the car but hate the seat.

Carrying Around Your "Bundle of Joy"

The Mount Sinai Sports Therapy Center in New York City offers this wrist-saving advice to new parents:

- When holding your baby, keep your hand and forearm aligned rather than bending at the wrist. Put a pillow on your lap to position the baby.
- Bend your knees, rather than your wrists, to lift the baby.
- When bathing a baby, use a bathtub ring or foam insert instead of holding the child.
- Use a baby pack whenever possible.
- Use both arms to support the baby.
- When pushing strollers, avoid bending your wrist or gripping the stroller handles.

Before you buy a new car, rent or borrow the same model. Spending five or ten minutes sitting in the driver's seat will not give you the same idea of the car's comfort as actually spending several days on the road in traffic. Your car should have power steering, an automatic rather than a stick shift, and a tiltable steering wheel.

When driving, Dr. Markison advises angling the steering wheel toward your lap and holding your hands at the four o'clock and eight o'clock positions instead of two and ten, which is too high. Avoid gripping the wheel forcefully.

AIRPLANES

When the gate agent asks for people who need extra time to pre-board the plane, get in line. Ask airline personnel or fellow passengers to help you stow your luggage.

Air travel will be more tolerable if you construct an ergonomic

---

RSI Wish List

The next time someone asks you what you want for Christmas, your birthday, or other special occasions, use this opportunity to ask for something that will be a hand saver. Small items—such as an electric stapler or pencil sharpener—are inexpensive. Big-ticket items such as telephone headsets or a high-quality computer chair may be possible if several people share the expense.

---

seat from the pillows in the overhead compartment. Request an aisle seat and—unless you experience turbulence—get up every twenty-five minutes to stretch and walk around the plane.

LUGGAGE

Many manufacturers make luggage with built-in wheels. Buy sturdy, *lightweight* luggage. One woman always took splints when she traveled to telegraph the fact that she needed help getting her baggage off the carousel.

By shipping items ahead, you can often significantly decrease the weight of your luggage. If you go home for the holidays, send gifts ahead. Same goes for books, hiking boots, and other heavy items.

9

RSI and Your Sex Life

While cohosting a seminar on coping with the challenges of RSI, a woman piped up from the rear of the room with a question that might have been on many people's minds, but which no one else dared ask: "The one thing you never talk about is sex! What are we supposed to do?"

Her query touched off an eruption of complaints, inquiries, and anecdotes. RSIers talked about everything from worrying about accidentally decapitating their partners with their splints to having trouble stating their needs.

RSI can seriously hamper your sex life. Expressing your sexuality in ways that are safe and comfortable for you is an important component to health regardless of your abilities. Many RSIers confess that having sex reduces symptoms; still, this area can present difficulties to people.

So, by popular request, here are some pointers. Remember, not every hint will apply to your circumstances, so choose what works for you.

Disability Does Not End Sexuality

You do not cease to be a loving, sensual being when your hands—or other parts of your body—become injured. In fact, far from being sexless, people with disabilities are often highly inventive about lovemaking and can have deeply satisfying experiences. While researching this chapter, I read case histories of people with other disabilities, hoping to find hints applicable to RSIers. A few of the people interviewed would be almost apologetic about their sexual experiences, saying things like, "Well, it might take us a couple of hours, but it's really great once we get there."

This is a problem?

Problems of Sexuality and Disability

Sexuality and disability can be a loaded combination. Depression, guilt, and feelings of shame, anxiety, or fear of increasing the injury may all lead to diminished sexual activity. Men with disabilities—especially combined with unemployment—may even experience impotence.

When men have limited or no mobility, they must rely on their partner to initiate sexual activity or prepare them physically, note the authors of *A Man's Guide to Coping with Disability.* "For men who value their role as the dominant partner in a sexual relationship, such a role reversal may be difficult, causing psychological distress and possibly avoidance of sexual activity. The role reversal may be equally difficult for the partner," they add.

Some women might have other concerns. It is not uncommon for a woman with RSI to be reluctant to get pregnant for fear of the physical strain of caring for a child. This concern may be difficult for a man who wants children to accept, and the relationship might suffer.

Dating with RSI

Having repetitive strain injury presents dating problems for a number of reasons. Samantha D. confessed to feeling bad because her boyfriend wanted her to play tennis and go skiing. "I wouldn't—and couldn't—do any of that." They broke up, for other reasons.

She also dated a physician for a month. "He was much more considerate," she said, "but . . . the one time he saw my arms swollen, he was shocked. I had carried groceries. Most of the time, I felt like he was humoring me—and this was a doctor."

People who feel rejected by lovers because of their injury may be reluctant to get involved again, fearing a repeat of this situation. Said Samantha D., "I'm nervous about getting involved with some-

Falling in Love

Falling in love is one of the best things that can happen to anyone at any time, but it is especially useful if you are injured. Problems do not seem to matter as much then; besides, you have someone with whom to share them. You don't worry as much. You feel better physically. In fact, I highly recommend that if you haven't already fallen in love you do so at the first opportunity. Unfortunately, I have found no surefire formula to meet the love of your life; Cupid, that prankster, strikes when (and targets those) you least expect.

Philosophers, poets, playwrights, and novelists have written about love for centuries. Anthropologists, biologists, and psychiatrists puzzle over it. Lyricists and mothers advise.

Love seems to have a mind and logic of its own. We

one else. I go to the doctor's two times a week. I see how it affects my mood. I'm twenty-eight and I feel like I have the problems of a ninety-year-old. I have to keep warm, wear layers. For someone who doesn't understand, it seems like you're being too fussy and hypochondriacal."

There is also the issue of sharing chores. "RSI presents a strain," she said. "You feel like you can't carry your own weight doing simple things like grocery shopping or putting up curtains. It's hard when the other person isn't being supportive. It's odd—I get a lot more support from friends."

The worst part may be the self-doubt you might feel about your own desirability. Samantha asked, "Who wants to be involved with someone who keeps running to doctors or who has a chronic problem?"

humans fall in love with people we can't have. People we loathe fall madly in love with us. We love the wrong people; we do not care. We make fools of ourselves over someone we later wonder how on earth we could have wanted. We swear eternal love to people we later betray, and are abandoned by lovers who vowed they would never leave. Our hearts break, we vow we will never love again, and then we meet someone new and the cycle begins again. A friend of mine once observed that love is completely irrational and unpredictable. "Of course, that's why everyone wants to do it so much," she said, laughing.

According to Dr. Markison, the key to finding love is to relax. This is because we probably tend to be more receptive to love in this state, and others find relaxed people easier to get close to and be around.

So relax—and I hope you fall in love!

Remember, being loved for yourself has nothing to do with your disability. Some people take the bull by the horns early on in their relationships. In a quiet moment, they will say something about their limitations, such as, "Are you going to be okay with this?" Your partner's reaction will reveal much about her or him, and the potential of a relationship.

RSI: THE ACID TEST

In a way, RSI can be a blessing, because by communicating your limitations to potential mates, you will get a very good sense of their character.

If someone persistently ignores your needs despite your attempts to educate him or her, that person is not a good choice. On the other hand, if someone encourages and accepts your frank communications for assistance, this person shows the kind of loving consideration that makes for a good life partner.

So do not be dismayed if someone rejects your injury; keep looking until you find the right person.

Ten Ways to a Better Sex Life

Sex is one area where you are likely to throw caution about your hands to the wind. Be careful not to strain your hands.

If you worry about accidentally whacking your partner with your splint in bed, talk to your doctor or occupational therapist about a softer splint. (See "Sleeping," page 119.)

COMMUNICATE WITH YOUR PARTNER

Being able to talk about problems is perhaps the most important factor in having a satisfying sex life. If you cannot communicate your needs, you are defeated before you begin. Your partner may not realize that certain things are risky, painful, or difficult for you now, so you need to explain that.

Maxwell S. attributed overcoming sexual problems to good communication between himself and his wife, Marie. He succeeded, he said, "because we talked, because I let her know what was happening with me, because I said, 'I can't do anything more with my hands tonight.'"

What should you say? Try, "I'm sorry, honey, but I can't do that right now. Can we do something else?" or, as Max S. sometimes says, "It's time for you to take over." By offering to do something else to please your partner, you show that you care. You're also giving your partner an opportunity to state her or his needs.

VIEW SEXUALITY AS A CONTINUUM

Many people feel like failures in bed because they focus solely on performance and achievement. But sexuality can be quite broad— from gazing into someone's eyes to full-blown lovemaking.

"Orgasm is a lot less important to me than it was when I was eighteen," said Max. "To me, the most important thing is hugging my wife, feeling my body gliding next to hers, smelling her smell, and knowing that she cares for me and I care for her. That's extremely sensual."

EXPERIMENT WITH SEXUAL AIDS

"A feather can be a devilish instrument of delight," Max reports. "It doesn't take much effort, and you can use your whole arm to use it."

Massage lotion intensifies sensations so you can employ a lighter touch. Use your fingertips to avoid strain on wrists.

You may never have considered using sex toys until now, but hands-free sexual aids are available for both men and women. Many couples enjoy experimenting with them.

If you do not feel comfortable shopping at retail stores, you can shop by mail. Some of the catalogs have helpful explanations about how sex toys work, as well as books and tapes about different aspects of sexuality.

USE YOUR WHOLE BODY

Lovemaking, especially foreplay, can be taxing on the hands and forearms. Max discovered that toes, knees, and shins can be used, too. In the beginning, he recalled, there was some laughter and awkwardness. "For one thing, using your toes gives you a different view. It feels different. But what was most important is that Marie knew I was in tune with her and doing what I could to give her pleasure."

Many people of both sexes also enjoy oral sex.

SOLO SEX IS AN OPTION

"Self-pleasuring is a primary source of sexual release for many single people and a regular part of many married couples' sex lives. It is a normal, natural form of expression," said Howard Ruppel, executive director of the American Association of Sex Educators, Counselors and Therapists.

If you can no longer do something for your partner, you might encourage him or her to take the initiative. When Steve T.'s wife did just that, he said, "Initially I felt I had failed her. On the other hand, she seemed to be having a good time." Now, however, it is something they both enjoy. "It is a definite turn-on for a man," he added.

INDULGE YOUR SEXUAL FANTASIES

As Ken Kroll and Erica Levy Klein, the authors of *Enabling Romance,* point out, a man or woman with a disability can still experience a degree of sexual fulfillment through fantasy when neither partnered nor solo sex is possible. "[F]antasy can soothe, comfort and make life more tolerable under even the most difficult circumstances."

ADVICE FOR MEN

If it hurts to put weight on your wrist, avoid the missionary position. Try putting the weight on your forearm instead (unless you have a nerve injury at the elbow). Experiment with a variety of positions until you find ones that are comfortable for you and your mate.

ADVICE FOR WOMEN

If making fast strokes hurts or tires your hands, you can ask your partner to put a hand over yours, and to make the movements for you. Many women may assume men want fast, firm, or hard pressure during foreplay, but do not realize the pleasures that can be obtained from varying pressure and speed. One man confessed that he far preferred it when a woman used a soft, slow touch.

READ ALL ABOUT IT

You and your partner may never have felt the need to read books on sexuality until you developed RSI; however, there are many excellent sexual guides that may give you ideas to try together. (See Resources and Further Reading, pages 223 and 231.)

SEEKING PROFESSIONAL HELP

Many people would not dream of asking their doctor for sexual advice. For that matter, many doctors may prefer not to hear about their patients' sexual problems. If you think a question about sexuality might trigger a sudden coughing fit or violent blush from your physician, see a licensed, qualified sex counselor or therapist. However, you may need to educate your sex therapist about RSI.

RSI Can Bring You Closer Together

Max reported feeling unmanly when he first injured his hands. "Making repetitive motions, the kind you do when you're making love, hurt me," he said. However, when he began to experiment with other techniques, he recaptured his sense of participation. Because of his wife's receptivity, an experience that might have been traumatic turned into an adventure for the two of them. "Marie is wonderfully understanding. She didn't make me feel like a failure," he said.

10
BEYOND ERGONOMICS: SOLVING COMMON WORK-RELATED PROBLEMS

Work issues present some of the thorniest challenges to healing from RSI. Many people endure job-related injuries, yet they want to continue working to bring in a paycheck. However, the productivity of the working injured may drop considerably if they comply with their doctor's orders to take regular breaks and stop painful activity. While quitting a job may be unthinkable, trying to keep up at the old pace may push them farther into pain and disability.

You should have a serious conversation with your doctor about whether to stay on the job. Remember: If you continue making repetitive movements with your hands and spending prolonged periods in static postures, you risk further damage. You are using injured tissue, which is not as strong as healthy tissue, so utmost attention must be paid to posture, pacing, and technique to prevent further damage to your musculature. With modifications to your workstation, careful technique and pacing, and a reduced workload, you might be able to work safely. You will also need the full backing of your employer and coworkers in order to protect yourself from flare-ups.

This is a tall order. One of the biggest complaints RSIers have is that they cannot keep up with workload.

Returning to Work After Rehabilitation

Many RSIers stop working to give their hands a rest, assuming that after they come back to work they will continue as before. They become very dismayed when they discover that after several relatively symptom-free weeks or months away from the job, their hands hurt within minutes of resuming work.

The trouble is, by the time many RSIers decide to rest their injury, much damage has already been done. Rest really helps prevent chronic injury when the symptoms of RSI still are quite subtle, but at that point most people have no idea they are injured.

"Injuries to soft tissue begin as a slight irritation," said Dr. Cianca. "As that injury develops, the swelling will increase. Pain will begin to set in and become longer and longer lasting. Typically, pain abates after people stop the activity. Then the pain may last a little bit longer even after stopping. In a stage-four–type injury, the pain is almost continuous. It doesn't disappear before that activity is engaged in again, so that you have an ongoing process of pain and inflammation.

"On a cellular level—at least in a first-time injury that's acute and less than a few weeks old—that process can be reversed, if proper steps are taken." Those steps include curtailing the offending activity, allowing the tissue to recover, and having some treatment if needed. If these signals are ignored, in some conditions, such as lateral epicondylitis (tennis elbow), the chronic condition actually results in a tendon-type tissue that is not functional. "It's poorly organized, it's not elastic, it just doesn't work well, and it serves as a continual irritant," said Dr. Cianca. "If that tissue is removed, people tend to do better, but again, you're never back to where you were before the injury. That's the long-term implication of those kinds of injuries."

There is a critical window of time during which reversal of soft tissue injury is possible, which is why denial of the problem in its early stages is such a problem. In addition to denial, said Dr. Cianca, "people are more concerned about getting the job done and their position with the firm. They don't allow themselves the luxury— rather than the right—to heal. We are not putting our priorities where they ought to be."

Unfortunately, by waiting for so long before they get into treatment, their injury becomes chronic. Now the damaged tissue is more susceptible to reinjury, and the relapse/healing/relapse cycle begins.

You may only be able to do half of your previous workload in order to preserve your hands. Restraining yourself from doing more than you should requires steely resolve. But the alternative is suffering a relapse that is worse than your initial injury, and continued loss of function in crucial daily activities.

Protecting Your Hands at Work: Tips for the Working Injured

AVOID USING COMPUTERS WHENEVER POSSIBLE

Because computer use gives rise to so many risk factors for RSI, it is better to avoid them entirely when possible. People who use computers for a living are rightly concerned about the lack of safer alternatives. But RSIers with other hand-intensive occupations can do themselves a huge favor by staying off the Internet and programs that create unnecessary computer work, such as computerized address books or checkbook-balancing systems.

USE SHORTCUTS

Look for ways to reduce keystrokes, such as using macros and quick keys. Keys can also be reconfigured to perform other functions. One man avoided the mouse by positioning the cursor with his trackball and "clicking" with the number 5 key. Talk to the technical support staff if you do not know how to use these features yourself.

AVOID OVERSTRESSING YOUR HANDS DURING LEISURE TIME

Many people do not take leisure-time activities into consideration when they tally up their daily hand use, and consequently underestimate their total hand allowance. This is not to say you must give up hobbies such as playing guitar or knitting entirely, but you should realize recreational hand use combines with occupational use, subjecting your hands to a high degree of stress.

Cynthia Z., a freelance editor in New York City, suspects that her habit of playing Solitaire on the computer contributed to her injury.

"I played Solitaire for three hours at a shot," she recalled. "It's addictive. People think, 'Oh, I'll just play one game'; then at 2 A.M. they bag it and wonder why their hand is in spasm the next day."

Video games are especially worrisome. Steve Greenlee, a former editor for a computer game magazine, said it is not uncommon for enthusiasts to start a game Friday night and play straight through until Sunday morning.

KEEP YOUR BODY FIT FOR WORK

If you are performing repetitive movements at work, it is your responsibility to keep your body strong and flexible enough to perform these highly taxing motions (see chapter 7, "The Healing Power of Exercise and Good Posture"). Be sure you warm up properly before you begin, and that your hands are warm while you are working.

TAKE FREQUENT BREAKS

Frequent, *regular* breaks are critical to preventing reinjury. "You cannot continually exceed your physical capacity, which lessens with injury," warned Dr. Cianca.

Do not allow yourself to work to the point of pain. Take a break as often as you need to, but certainly well *before* you feel any symptoms of strain, such as fatigue, soreness, tingling, or even hyperawareness of your hands. If you wait—or work in pain—you will be causing damage to the soft tissue. This advice also applies to people who say they do not type much, because static loading is such a big contributing factor to RSI.

For the self-employed or managers, this advice is somewhat easier to put into practice—*if* you can exercise the necessary discipline to stop working when you have reached your limit.

Work habits can be deeply ingrained, as Gary Karp knows. When he was starting out, he said, "I had a blast working sixteen hours a day, much of it at the computer. It was exciting, it was fun. You can only do that for so long, but you get in the habit of working at that pace." Although Gary is now self-employed, he said, "To this day I find it hard to work at the computer in a relaxed mode, because I spent all those years with constant deadline, detail-intensive work."

Many creative people fear losing momentum or ideas if they stop. But ideas don't die. They keep coming back until you put them down on paper. So don't worry; you won't lose anything.

For many employees, breaks are either tacitly verboten, or they *think* they will be punished for taking a breather. Kate M. said, "I have a message that pops up every twenty minutes to tell me to take a break. I just keep hitting the Return button to get it off my screen. You get caught in these deadlines. In the back of my mind, I keep thinking, 'If I don't keep it up, I won't have a job.' "

Many people play computer games during their break, but that's not a good idea. You would be better off getting up, doing some upper-body stretches, and taking a short walk. If stretching in public makes you self-conscious, go to a private area or close your office door.

Do not wait for your timer to go off before taking a break if you have symptoms. Let your body guide you.

As noted earlier, some people are afraid even to look away from the screen for a few minutes to rest their eyes for fear of being accused of malingering. Please bear in mind that your reluctance to take breaks may have more to do with your own work ethic than company policy. Many employers fully understand the need for regular breaks. If you have doubts, have a heart-to-heart talk with your employer.

PACE YOURSELF

Pacing differs from taking breaks, because it refers to how much work you do during a given day as well as the length of time between hand-intensive sessions. The lack of self-pacing is one of the leading risk factors for RSI. When left to their own devices, people work in fits and starts; when they have had enough, they call it a day. For instance, if you were painting a wall and you got tired, you would most likely stop. Such self-regulation is not possible in many job settings.

Rather, people are evaluated on the basis of how much work they produce during a given amount of time. So if you are expected to execute a minimum number of keystrokes per hour, this external pacing system may be your nemesis if you cannot keep up with the pace.

This is particularly challenging in professions that require "real-time" work. As Bob Hubbard, an oboist, pointed out, dancers, musicians, and surgeons work in real time. "The actual performance starts now, goes at this pace, then it's done. There's no time to revise. You can't stop a symphony and say, 'I need a break.' "

AVOID SITTING FOR LONG PERIODS

To counteract the adverse effects of sitting, stand as often as possible during the day. Get into the habit of standing when the phone rings. Don't be angry if the call interrupts you in the middle of a project; be glad you have a reason to stand.

KEEP BREATHING

It has been my observation that computer users tend to hold their breath, especially when they are waiting for files or graphics to download. To my knowledge, there have been no formal studies on this phenomenon, but other computer users say they have noticed this tendency in themselves.

The Walking Trick

The next time you're stuck on a project, instead of puzzling things out in your chair, go for a walk—preferably in fresh air. Walking brings blood to the brain, and the solution to your problem often comes to you as you stroll.

Also, do all your meetings really have to take place sitting in a conference room? If not, ask your colleague to join you and have the meeting while you walk.

Holding your breath or breathing shallowly is a bad practice, because your muscles need oxygen to work properly. Shallow breathing tightens the muscles around the neck, which can lead to nerve compression.

THINGS TO DO WHEN YOU DOWNLOAD

Computer users often become frustrated when programs run slowly. Instead of fuming because the graphics are taking too long to download, use the time as an opportunity to get up out of your chair and move. Breathe from your belly. Do your neck stretches. Don't stare at the screen while nothing is happening—look out the window and relax your eyes.

The Proper Workstation

People often do not appreciate the damage a poor setup can do to their body until they are injured. Self-employed people sometimes say they cannot afford to buy a good computer chair or other hand-saving accessories. The same people generally find the money to make these purchases after spending several thousand dollars on physical therapy and doctor's visits. People are often very disappointed to discover that new furniture does not take away their pain.

A similar thing happens with many people who work for companies. All too often, by the time people finally receive the ergonomic equipment they need, they lose their jobs anyway because they are too disabled to work.

WHO PAYS?

A friend of mine related the following all-too-common experience when he started at a new job. "You should see my new computer! It is so fast, it has all kinds of software, and it is permanently connected to the Internet," he raved. However, he added, "If you could see my workstation, you'd need CPR! I spent half the day trying to adjust my chair. It was horrendous!"

Some companies spend thousands of dollars on computer hardware and software but refuse to buy adjustable furniture and equipment.

Employees get very inventive about solving these problems when management is slow to respond. One trader became so frustrated that his company would not provide him with a telephone headset that he bought one himself—and submitted the bill with his travel and entertainment expenses! But some companies do not allow people to spend their *own* money on proper chairs because it would be against company policy.

Everyone Needs a Good Chair

The chair is so critical to comfort and safety that one wonders why *all* chairs are not "ergonomic" (i.e., safe, adjustable, and comfortable). Surely if manufacturers put a little thought into designing better chairs, they could design models within everyone's budget. It is also puzzling that employers often are willing to buy good chairs only for people who are "having problems" (e.g., severe back, neck, or arm pain). It would be to everyone's benefit if all employees in a company were comfortable at work.

THE GOLDILOCKS POSTULATE:
FINDING A CHAIR THAT FITS

If you wore a size ten shoe, you wouldn't try to cram your foot into a size five. By the same token, people come in all shapes and sizes, and as Goldilocks wisely observed, they need Mama Bear–, Papa Bear–, and Baby Bear–size chairs.

Some corporate policies are at odds with this common sense, however. Marlene Green, who owns an ergonomics accessories company, knows firsthand that for people who work in corporations, how a chair looks is often more important than how a chair feels. She told me the following story:

"There was a very big guy who worked in the back office," said Green. "So they bought him an extra-large chair." Big guy, big chair—makes sense, right?

Apparently the higher-ups were concerned because his chair was different from everyone else's, Green explained. "They took

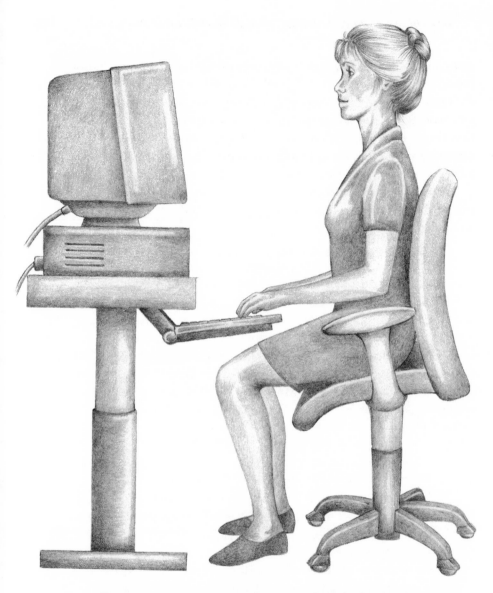

To set up your computer workstation, adjust the height of the chair so that your feet are resting flat on the floor. If your feet don't reach the floor, use a footrest. Tilt the seat so your hips are slightly higher than your knees; position the backrest to support your lower back. Lower the keyboard tray until your upper arms and forearms form a 90-degree angle or slightly greater. Place the monitor an arm's length away from your torso, your eyes level with the top of the screen. Copyholders should be placed at monitor level.

Note that the hands of the figure in the illustration are floating above the keyboard in neutral position.

away the chair that made him comfortable and gave him the same model that everyone else had, so all the chairs would look the same. Everyone had to sit in the same chair no matter how big you are."

Meanwhile, the now-uncomfortable employee anguished in an ill-fitting seat, while a chair that fit him languished in storage. If a company desires a uniform look, why not use the same upholstery fabric to cover appropriate chairs?

People may think that overly soft executive chairs make a more powerful impression on clients. But comfort and injury prevention should be the main criteria, not status.

Desk Accessories

THE FOOTREST

Your chair should adjust low enough for you to rest your feet flat on the floor. If you are short, and your feet dangle, this can create back pain and cut off the circulation to the lower leg. If you cannot adjust the chair to the right height, ask the chair manufacturer if a shorter pedestal is available. Otherwise, you can support your feet with a footrest.

THE KEYBOARD SUPPORT

An adjustable keyboard surface is critical for safety, because if you must raise your elbows to type or use the mouse, you place enormous strain on your upper body.

When choosing a keyboard support, consider several factors:

- Is it easy to adjust? If it is not, you will be less likely to adjust it.
- Does it roll smoothly out of the way or does it bump and jerk?
- Is it made of sturdy material, or does it quiver and shake while you work? An unstable surface can add unnecessary physical tension.
- What is the underside of the support like? Do your knees and thighs constantly bump into knobs and levers? Does the un-

The Elements of Proper Seating

Here are some guidelines for choosing the proper chair, but remember that you should spend as much time as possible *not* sitting in it!

THE CHAIR SEAT

The seat (or seatpan, in office-furnishing parlance) should be firm but not hard. The front edge of the chair should slope slightly so it does not cut into your thigh, and there should be enough room for you to put a loose fist between your knee and the front of the seat.

The seatpan should also tilt so that the pelvis is slightly higher than the knees. This reduces strain on the lower back.

THE BACKREST

For computer work, the backrest should support the spine in an erect position. Chairs that give way when you sit back lead to craned necks. If you like to recline while you think, get a backrest that can lock in place *or* tilt back.

ARMRESTS

Armrests actually support the shoulder, allowing you to relax the muscles around the neck. They should be short enough to let you come close to your desk or keyboard, adjustable so you do not have to slouch or hunch your shoulders to reach them, and padded if you have nerve problems.

Some people object to armrests altogether because they get in the way while they're working or because they use them to support their arms while using the mouse or keyboard. If this is the case for you, you might be able to remove them.

derside have rough or sharp edges that will ruin women's hosiery?

• Keyboard trays that slope downward, toward the knee in "negative tilt," are intended to help people avoid the position of dorsiflexion. Dorsiflexion is bending the wrist so the top of the hand moves upward, as in the position of your hands if the wrists rest on the table during typing, or of a crossing guard halting traffic. Do not counteract negative tilt by raising the kickstand on the back of the keyboard.

PLACEMENT OF EQUIPMENT

Computer equipment is frequently plopped any old way on the nearest horizontal surface. From then on, people contort their bodies around it instead of moving the heavy, bulky hardware closer to them. Some computer users will sit with keyboards way off to one side for hours instead of simply sliding the keyboard in front of them. People often react to the suggestion they move the keyboard or adjust their chair by saying, "Oh, I'm only going to be here a second." Seconds turn into minutes and hours, and meanwhile the body suffers.

You wouldn't drive in a car if you hadn't adjusted the car seat. Do not sit in a workstation that has not been properly adjusted.

Keyboards and Voice Systems

SPLIT KEYBOARDS

Standard keyboards force most people to wing their elbows or ulnar deviate their wrists. Ulnar deviation is the bent angle of the wrists as they reach sideways, such as to strike the Shift, Enter, or Tab key. Split keyboards get around this problem, because you can adjust the keyboard instead of twisting your wrists. But be sure to get a keyboard that splits in two separate pieces, not one molded into shape, unless your body happens to fit that design.

VOICE-ACTIVATED SOFTWARE

Voice-activated software has often been hailed as the solution to repetitive strain injuries. It would be wonderful if this were so; but unfortunately it is not, for many reasons.

The human body works best when you can use many muscle groups at a task, preferably in a stop-and-start fashion. When you force the entire body to remain still—static loading—while you rely entirely on a small muscle, you set the stage for injury.

Repetition, another risk factor, comes into play if you rely on the voice to do all the work. If you don't take frequent breaks, the vocal muscles can become sore and irritated—and can become seriously injured. Sometimes the term "vocal cords" (which are called "vocal folds" in medical circles) confuses people, noted Lynda Marvin, a speech pathologist and assistant professor in the Speech and Hearing Department of Long Island University. "When you say 'cords,' they think they have strings in their throats like violins," she explained. In fact, they are actually more like lips—fleshy folds made up of muscle, connective tissue, and mucous membrane.

Many voice programs require discrete speech, which means that instead of speaking conversationally, you must say each word separately. This is very hard on the voice.

Gary Karp, who uses a voice-activated system, said, "My neck gets very sore from voice dictation. You're completely frozen. You don't even get to use your arms." Karp deliberately moves his head during saves and does light editing with his hands.

Perhaps someday people will have the option of combining keyboard and vocal commands, which would lessen the strain on both the voice and the hands.

Voice-activated programs are a godsend when they allow people to work, but remember to employ safe technique (see page 178).

SCANNERS

There is no justification for a human hand entering data when a machine can do it. If you frequently type new input from copy, purchase a good scanner.

TELEPHONE HEADSETS

Headsets are essential for both preventing and coping with injury. Many RSIers need one because holding the telephone is tiring or it makes their hands fall asleep.

Cradling the telephone receiver with the shoulder puts the neck in an awkward position and stresses the surrounding muscles. This can lead to serious injury. You don't realize how much you cradled the phone until you get a telephone headset and find that your hands are wondrously free—to riffle through files, to pick up a book or catalog, or to write—*without* neck strain.

The following points should be taken into consideration when purchasing a headset:

- You need to decide whether you want a commercial-grade or retail headset. Commercial-grade headsets are designed for people who are on the phone many hours a day. They tend to be well designed, comfortable, and sturdy. Retail headsets, such as those purchased in electronics stores, cost less but can break more easily and deliver inferior sound and comfort.

    If you care about durability, comfort, and the quality of sound—not just what you hear but also what your caller hears—choose a commercial-grade headset.
- Headsets that fit neatly around the ear are good for people who dislike headbands. But if you wear glasses, this may not be a good choice because of the extra weight on your ear.
- Some headsets have one earpiece; others have two. The latter, known as binaural headsets, help people in noisy environments hear the other party better. High-end models even have noise-canceling microphones, which transmit your voice without background noise.
- Cordless headsets give you the most freedom to stand and walk during telephone conversations. (During winter months, be careful not to touch anything that might give you a static shock during a conversation, or you may temporarily lose your phone connection. You won't actually lose the call, because your handset will still be off the hook, but you won't be able to hear your caller because of static. Just tell your party

what happened using the handset, readjust the headset, and go back to your conversation.)

Cordless headsets emit a weak electromagnetic field. Joseph Salvatore, M.D., director of the National Registry for the Health Effects of Nonionizing Radiation, said there is no strong data to suggest that this causes malignancy. "The risk is minor," said Louis Slesin, editor of *Microwave News* in New York City, "but it is another source." So consider this factor in your decision.

• Before making your purchase, you should find out about return policies. There is a world of difference between reading catalog copy and actually using a product. If a headset slips, pinches, or irritates you, you probably won't use it.

TELEPHONE DIALING SYSTEMS

For RSIers who have trouble dialing the phone as well as holding one to their ear—or who must enter a lot of numbers so calls can be billed to clients—programmable dialing and voice dialing are essential (see page 128).

Cautions About Risky Devices

WRIST RESTS

Wrist rests can create big problems. "The weight of the upper extremity, from the shoulder down, is resting on the wrist," pointed out Dr. Piligian. By doing this, you immobilize the shoulders. "They may already be tired, on their way to a frank or recognizable injury." Now the fingers and wrist must deviate even more from neutral position to perform typing and computing movements.

You should be using your own muscles to hold up your arms; if they fatigue, you should rest them rather than propping them up with arm or wrist rests. Wrist rests do provide a soft surface to lay your hands on when you are *not* typing.

LAPTOP COMPUTERS

Laptop computers have several inherent problems. If you put the laptop where the screen falls within proper viewing range, the keyboard is too high. Put the keyboard at the right level for the hands, and the neck must bend to see the screen. Either way, the upper body is at risk for injury. Not only that, the built-in trackballs are sometimes very stiff, and they can overburden the thumb. Laptops are also heavy, especially when combined with a briefcase and luggage. In addition, business travelers often work on surfaces that are too high, or airplane tray tables that are very confining.

In short, laptops present too many hazards that cannot be obviated with careful positioning and good technique. Unless you can plug the laptop into a standard monitor—or use the laptop monitor with a separate keyboard—so you can place *both* items at appropriate levels, do not use one. Do not work with it on your lap, and avoid using the built-in input device.

THE MOUSE TRAP

When the mouse was first introduced, it was designed to make computer software easier to use. Instead of memorizing key combinations, all you had to do was point and click. Software designers embraced this concept, and mouse-driven programs multiplied. However, when you look at some risk factors for repetitive strain injuries—usually a combination of repetition, force, awkward positioning, and poor technique—several problems become obvious.

First of all, where do you put it? Even if you have a tray, often there is not room for both mouse and keyboard, so many people put it on the desk, which is both too high and too far away. This position can lead to strain from the fingers all the way to the neck and shoulder.

Then consider repetition. The keyboard lets you distribute the work between two hands, relieving the burden on the dominant hand. With the mouse, you repeatedly use one hand to position, click, and drag the cursor.

Not only does the mouse overwork the dominant hand; it also overworks the click finger. Instead of using both hands, the index finger of one hand usually does all the work. To compound the problem, many people use far more force than necessary to click. They may also be holding the mouse in a death grip for long periods.

Your dominant hand performs a multitude of daily tasks, such as writing, opening doors, and buttering bread. This adds up, especially with several hundred mouse clicks thrown in. You begin to appreciate just how much you depend on your dominant hand when it becomes painful to use a Touch-Tone phone or punch your code into the automatic teller machine.

There is also the design of the mouse, which fits more or less into the hollow of the hand. Most people plant their wrists and forearms on the desk while they position the cursor with waves of the wrist. This action bends the wrist upward and sideways at the same time, placing a tremendous strain on the forearm muscles. Also, instead of allowing you to instinctively use the powerful muscles in your back and shoulder—as typewriters do—the mouse encourages you to rely on the delicate muscles in your fingers and forearms.

Finally, mice can be very hard to control. Sometimes the cursor skates off the screen, and you have to hold the click button down while you lift and reposition the mouse. When this happens, you tend to grip the mouse, thereby straining the muscles in your arm. You can use good technique to help position the mouse, but you are still faced with the click and drag.

Are trackballs, styluses, or touchpads any safer? The answer is no. A trackball, like a mouse, puts the hand in an awkward position and requires the use of the dominant hand and thumb. People also tend to flatten, rather than curve, their fingers when using a trackball, and this contraction of the muscles can lead to forearm strain. Touchpads are no improvement. Once again, they overuse the dominant hand, and people tend to flatten their fingers while using them, which strains and exhausts the muscles. They are also sometimes slow to respond and require heavy finger pressure to operate. Styluses can be very troublesome because improper handwriting habits are often much harder to change than poor computing technique.

As you can see, one-handed input devices should be avoided

altogether or used sparingly. (See page 173 for some pointers on mouse-free maneuvering.)

The Interpersonal Aspects of Work

TALKING TO YOUR BOSS

Getting your boss to understand your limitations can be very difficult for some RSIers. Kate M. said, "My boss says, 'You're not supposed to be on the computer,' then she'll turn around and give me several new jobs that have to be done on the computer." This kind of double message is as infuriating as it is counterproductive.

April S. also experienced problems in this regard. "The foreman used to say, 'Are you done? Are you done?' I yelled, 'Stop pushing me!' But I continued to work."

Many people are expected to work at maximum speed every day. From some employers' point of view, every moment you are not productive is money down the drain. Employees would generally rather be working all the time, too—either because of their own work ethic or because they don't want their superiors to think they are slacking off.

But you must not push beyond your limits. As Sylvie Erb said, "It is difficult to confront your boss and say, 'This is how much I can do today.' But what is more important, your boss or your body?"

TALKING TO YOUR COWORKERS

Depending on their attitude, coworkers can be a big help or hindrance in your ability to continue your job. One office worker said, "If I can't carry my load at work, it's okay." She knew she could depend on coworkers to help out.

Other RSIers are not so fortunate. They overhear snide remarks about "people who are not pulling their weight." If this is the case with you, and you cannot resist the peer pressure to overwork, you should become more assertive or find another job.

Do not allow yourself to be bullied out of your breaks. Otherwise, you risk worsening the injury.

PROBLEMS OF THE SELF-EMPLOYED

Despite their autonomy in certain areas, self-employed people experience many of the same problems as salaried employees, and then some. For one thing, the work frequently comes in chunks with immediate deadlines, instead of a steady stream that would allow proper pacing. They often work without any help, too. Like employees, independent contractors can be afraid to stop for a break. "I pushed myself over the limit so many times," said April S. "I wanted to please my client. I had my reputation to worry about. You hate to say no, hate to disappoint someone."

The specter of no work haunts the self-employed. "I went through the recession. Back then, three days of work a week were wonderful," April recalled. "It's not stable. It's everything or nothing. I never could pace myself."

Your Job or Your Hands

Over and over, people have made the point that they could continue their jobs, *provided they could work at their own pace.* As rational as this sounds on paper, it is not always easy in practice.

You simply may not be able to put in more than two or three hours at the computer (or other repetitive movement). From your employer's point of view, this may be unacceptable. Some employers do not understand that retrofitting a workstation will not bring an employee's former productivity level back. From the company's point of view, limiting a worker's computer time is asking for too much, especially after the firm spent several hundred dollars refurbishing the employee's workstation. In addition, only so many people are going to be hired to do a set amount of work.

The pressure to produce can also come from within. Many RSIers feel they cannot refuse work or rest when they need it. But remember, repetitive motions are part of what gave you your injury. If you continue that activity—as in computer use—you risk reinjuring yourself.

You must ask yourself what is more important to you: your job or your hands. This is a difficult question. As Dr. Piligian pointed out, "You want to try always to keep people working. But you have to remember that if they do not have use of their hands, that itself is going to preclude them from working, so you're defeating your own purpose. You are buying a little bit of time now, but you're going to lose that and more later."

THINK ABOUT AN ALTERNATIVE CAREER

Even if you are happily employed and believe you can do your job without injury, it is not a bad exercise to consider what you would do if for some reason this were not the case. In fact, over time RSI can get worse, simply because—careful technique and pacing notwithstanding—you are continuing an injurious activity. Thinking about a career change while you are securely employed is far easier than doing so with the wolf at the door.

QUITTING WHILE YOU'RE AHEAD

I can't tell you exactly when I knew the game was over, but I couldn't hold on to things and I was in pain all the time. I realized I was having symptoms of carpal tunnel syndrome. I thought, "If I have carpal tunnel now—on top of tendinitis, cubital tunnel syndrome, and thoracic outlet syndrome—if carpal tunnel doesn't convince me to quit, what will?"
—JANE H., an injured videotape editor

Many RSIers doggedly fight to keep their jobs for years, often suffering relapses, going out on disability, and coming back again only to incur new injuries that may be even worse. When every repetitive movement is agonizing, eventually there is no choice but to try to find an alternative job that does not strain your hands—or to give up work entirely.

Letting go of your job can be especially painful if you love what you do and it provides your major identity. For Jane H., the decision to quit her job took almost six years. "I would never have believed I would give up my career," said Jane. "I was one of the first women doing technical work in television, and I paid a high price. Younger women won't know what the first wave of women went through. People assumed you got coffee. Here I'd gone through holy hell to have a job I could be proud of, then I had to leave it, not because I couldn't do it, but because I couldn't *do* it.

"I made my decision by myself one afternoon. My boss was extremely supportive. They have never not believed me. They even engineered an adaptor to my equipment."

Despite these attempts to accommodate her, she said that "doing the simplest things, I was having burning pain." Saying good-bye was painful, too. "My boss said he was devastated. Everyone was in shock."

Your Legal Alternatives

WORKERS' COMPENSATION

If you are injured on the job, you are entitled to Workers' Compensation insurance, which can cover medical treatment, lost wages, and other benefits. In recent years, Workers' Compensation has been affected by the same kinds of cutbacks that have swept medical insurance and welfare. "While economists and Wall Street cheer market-driven care, patients grumble," wrote Steffie Woolhandler and David Himmelstein of Harvard Medical School in an article in the *American Journal of Public Health.* "HMO enrollees are more than twice as likely as fee-for-service patients to complain that care is not appropriate, that examinations are not thorough, and that physicians do not care enough or spend enough time."

If your Workers' Compensation claim is handled through your employer's HMO or PPO, another wrinkle is added to the problem. The insurance company can make you seek treatment only by certain approved doctors, said Dominick Tuminaro, a New York Workers' Compensation attorney. "These doctors are involved in a contractual relationship with an insurance carrier or employer, with the objective of saving money on care and Workers' Compensation benefits. If they don't produce savings, the business could go elsewhere," said Tuminaro. Doctors who spend enough time with patients to obtain a complete occupational medical history and perform a thorough examination may be branded "unprofitable" because they see fewer patients than do their colleagues. "Most managed-care contracts allow the firm to fire practitioners without cause," add Woolhandler and Himmelstein, and "job insecurity makes physicians toe the managed-care line." Managed-care insurers also impose "uniform" protocols and therefore can dictate the way your physician is allowed to treat your injury, such as limiting the number of physical therapy sessions you receive.

Several key decisions are made by the treating physician:

- Is this injury work-related?
- Are you disabled?
- If so, what is the degree of disability?
- Is the disability permanent?
- Is there a permanent impairment?

None of these questions have to do with treatment; they have to do with judgments about disability, which determines the money you will be awarded for your injury. And this, according to Tuminaro, is critical. If your doctor answers no to any of those questions, it could eliminate or reduce payment for lost income and/or medical treatment. You can ask for another opinion, but Tuminaro says second-opinion specialist panels are heavily staffed with doctors who have worked for insurance carriers and are likely to rule in favor of the employer and insurance carriers. You can pay out of pocket to see a physician of your choice, but Tuminaro fears that this will be perceived as "doctor shopping." Your physician may lose credibility because he or she is viewed by the judge as a hired gun.

A doctor can declare you temporarily totally, temporarily partially, permanently partially, or permanently totally disabled. These distinctions can mean a great deal to you. "Wage replacement for a temporarily totally disabled person might be $300 a week, whereas a partially disabled person may receive as little as $75, assuming an average weekly wage of $400," said Tuminaro.

Can you see your medical report? Yes, eventually. But unless your doctor is willing to provide you with a copy beforehand, you may have to wait until your next Workers' Compensation hearing to know what it contains.

Here is some advice:

- Seek the counsel of an experienced Workers' Compensation attorney (see Resources).
- File a claim as soon as you receive a medical diagnosis that the injury is work-related. *You do not have to be out of work to file.* Don't wait, because if you do, you may have to wait months to get wage-replacement benefits while you are out of work.
- It is not enough for your doctor to tell you to stay off the keyboard because it aggravates your injury; the doctor must state that the injury has been *caused* by the work you do.
- If you receive a notice that your claim has been controverted by your insurance carrier, that does *not* mean it has been denied. Talk to your attorney about what should happen next.
- Opt out of your HMO. Choose a treating physician who understands RSI and is willing to advocate on your behalf. Your physician should also understand the Workers' Compensation system, in order to fill out the forms properly.

USING THE AMERICANS WITH DISABILITIES ACT

Many people erroneously assume they are protected from losing their livelihood because of job-related injury by the Americans with Disabilities Act (ADA). This law is intended to protect individuals with disabilities from discrimination in employment, but unfortunately it does not necessarily help you keep your current job if you become disabled.

Under the ADA, employers are required to provide "reasonable accommodation" that would allow someone with a disability to perform the job. In the case of RSI, this might mean taking time off, modifying equipment, or reassignment to light-duty jobs. However, such accommodation is not required if it imposes an undue hardship on the employer's business (such as costing too much), and if a light-duty position is not available, the employer is not obligated to create one.

Sometimes employers will offer an injured employee a different position within the company. This may not be in your area of expertise, though, as was the case with two Florida journalists who were assigned to jobs patrolling the parking lot of their newspaper.

WORKERS' COMPENSATION VERSUS THE ADA

While Workers' Compensation laws provide compensation for work-related injuries, the ADA prohibits and punishes discrimination on account of an individual's disability. "If you want compensation for your injury, then you think about Workers' Compensation. If you want to return to work, the issue falls under the ADA," advised Richard Corenthal, a New York attorney who specializes in the ADA.

Filing a Workers' Compensation claim does not prevent an injured worker from filing a charge of discrimination under the ADA. However, some employers have raised defenses to ADA claims because an employee has filed a Workers' Compensation claim. They argue that an employee cannot claim to be injured and unable to work *while* claiming, under the ADA, to be qualified to perform the essential functions of the job. The key point here, according to Corenthal, is that under the ADA, the employer is required to provide reasonable accommodation. If an employer does not make reasonable accommodation, what choice does an employee have but to apply for Workers' Compensation?

Under the ADA, you can get reinstatement, back pay, compensatory and punitive damages, and attorney's fees if you win your case. However, litigation under the ADA has been difficult. It is very hard to prove discrimination, because employers may cite a reason unrelated to the disability for not hiring—or for firing—you.

THINK BEFORE YOU SUE

Lawsuits can be time-consuming, frustrating, and sometimes ultimately disappointing, so consider the issue carefully before you sue. "The best situation is if you never need to call a lawyer," said Corenthal.

FAMILY AND MEDICAL LEAVE ACT (FMLA)

[A]n eligible employee shall be entitled to a total of 12 work-weeks of leave during any 12-month period . . . because of a serious health condition that makes the employee unable to perform the functions of the position of such employee.
—SECTION 2612, Family and Medical Leave Act of 1993

The Family and Medical Leave Act of 1993 can be of great help to RSIers who need time to sort through their medical dilemmas. Under the FMLA, certain employers must grant up to twelve weeks of unpaid leave for health reasons. The law also provides that the employer must allow the employee to return to the same job and continue paying insurance premiums.

The FMLA can buy you time, because you will be able to stop the injurious activity and rest your injury, get medical advice, and make alternative plans. The FMLA does not cover every employee, so talk to an attorney to see if you qualify and find out how to follow proper procedures.

SOCIAL SECURITY DISABILITY

If you are unable to work because of your injury, you may qualify for Social Security Disability insurance. This government program is not intended for short-term, temporary, or partial disabilities. The disability must last for at least one year, but you do not have to wait a year to apply for benefits. You may file a claim as soon as a condition is disabling and a doctor can predict that it is expected to last a year, according to Barbara Kate Repa in her book, *Your Rights in the Workplace.* The amount of money you receive is based on your average income, which may be substantially lower after your injury. Note only that there is a waiting period of five months before you begin receiving payments.

Under current rules, if you are prevented from doing your current job but could still perform another kind of "substantial gainful" work—which Social Security defines as any job paying $500 a month or more—you will not qualify.

To apply for benefits, call the Social Security Administration office listed in the government section of the phone book.

——— 11 ———
PROPER TECHNIQUE AT WORK

Until they endure an injury, most people have no idea how important proper technique is. Technique refers to how you habitually use your hands during an activity. Without realizing it, many people repeatedly misuse their hands, making themselves vulnerable to injury. Faulty technique would not matter if you made only one or two movements sporadically, but when you spend hours on end using your hands, good technique can save your hands—and bad technique can induce severe injuries.

When you are in an inflammatory stage of injury, any use of the hand might hurt, so sometimes technique retraining must wait until pain subsides. This can sometimes take weeks or months. When you become pain-free. You will discover that proper technique will help keep pain away; conversely, going back to your old habits (or overdoing it!) will bring back pain and soreness.

When you begin to go back to the activity, you must control pain. This is accomplished by stopping the offensive activity *before* you feel symptoms. If you can type for twenty minutes without pain, stop every ten minutes and take a ten- to twenty-minute rest. If you are still sore, stop for the rest of the day and see how you feel the next morning.

Make sure your hands are warm before you commence the activity. Dr. Markison recommends the following test for hand temperature: Hold your hands to your cheek (the thermometer of the body). If they feel cool, warm them before you start.

Learning to use proper technique and posture can be difficult at first. When one man found out what he must do to type or play the piano correctly, he protested, "I can't remember all that! I've got a piece of music to play!"

But you can and must use proper posture and technique at all times. It is quite possible to focus on work and body awareness at the same time. It is even easier once you discover these techniques to reduce pain. It just takes practice.

Basic Computer Technique

KEEP YOUR HANDS IN NEUTRAL POSITION

When the hand is in neutral position, the middle knuckle and center of the wrist are in a straight line. The fingers curve, and the wrist is neither bent upward nor bent down. To find neutral, simply sit with your shoulders relaxed and let your arms hang by your side, fingers relaxed. Your hand will fall into neutral position naturally. Now, without changing the position of your wrists and fingers, bring your hands to the keyboard. The tops of the wrists should be held about 20 degrees from horizontal, the palms should be lifted toward each other about 30 degrees, with fingers relaxed and gently curved.

> • **Avoid dorsiflexion.** The minute you lift the top of your hand, you tense the forearm muscles. Instead, let your hands float over the keys, with straight wrists, moving the elbow to position the fingers. Do not rest your wrists on anything as you type.

> • **Avoid ulnar deviation.** Keep the middle knuckle in line with the center of the wrist as you move over the keys or use the mouse or trackball (see illustration, page 167). Do not twist the hand to reach peripheral keys such as Shift, Enter, or Control. Lift the whole hand, position a finger over the desired key, and then strike.

> • **Keep all your fingers curved.** Do not stretch your hands to reach two keys at once or a position above the row you are working on. Move the arm and position the finger over the key.

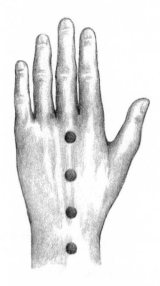

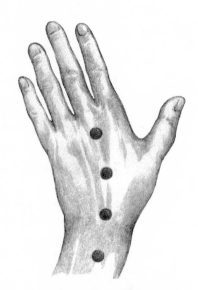

Neutral Wrist Position   **Ulnar Deviation**

Ulnar deviation refers to the bent angle of the wrists as they reach sideways for the Shift, Enter, or Tab key. This position places strain on the forearm. Instead, *move your whole hand* in neutral position over to the key and then strike. (See page 148 for a horizontal view of the neutral wrist.)

For commands that require two keystrokes at once, use both hands.

USE DOTS AS AN AID

To help yourself maintain your hands in a neutral position, buy some bright stick-on dots, such as those used to color-code files. Place one dot on the knuckle of the middle finger, one in the center of your wrist, and one along the axis of those points. The bright dots provide a visual cue to keep your hand in the proper position: All you have to do is line up the dots. You can instantly see when your hands are out of alignment.

There are all kinds of uses for the dots. People who point their pinkies and thumbs can use them as reminders to keep them down.

Sparing the Thumb

Rather than moving the thumb independently to strike the space bar, keep it relaxed and roll the whole hand until the thumb depresses the bar. Or avoid using the thumb altogether and use two strong fingers (index and middle) together to space.

DR. MARKISON'S TAPE TRICK

Dr. Markison uses this trick to teach patients to relax the thumb joint: Take some adhesive tape (the cloth kind doctors use is good, because it does not pull the skin) and place it across your thumb joint (see illustration, page 169). Now move your thumb up and down. If you hold your thumb too far up or down, the tape wrinkles. Practice typing with the tape on so you learn how it feels to keep the thumb relaxed as you work.

You can also write tiny reminders to "Breathe!" "Relax your thumb!" and "Stretch" and stick them to your monitor.

The dots are cheap, colorful, and easy to find. They come off easily, without pulling or gumming the skin. Buy a package in your favorite color, and use them to help you improve your technique.

PROS AND CONS OF HUNT-AND-PECK TYPING

Self-taught typists generally hunt and peck. This sidesteps two technique problems right away, because you generally avoid dorsiflexion and ulnar deviation.

Hunt-and-peck typing is not without risk, however. The heavy head hangs on the neck muscles as the typist searches for a key. In addition, some hunters type with their middle finger instead of

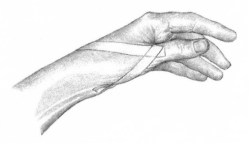

Dr. Markison's Tape Trick

Take two strips of cloth adhesive tape and place them in a V meeting at your second thumb joint. The bottom piece of tape should continue along the pad of muscle on the palm side of the thumb.

keeping all their fingers curved, which strains many muscles in the hand and forearm.

PUT TWO FINGERS ON WIDE KEYS

Instead of using your little finger to strike wide keys such as Enter, Shift, Control, or Alt, let it relax completely and use two fingers, such as the index and middle, or middle and ring fingers (being careful to keep *all* fingers curved).

This technique will slow you down, but when it comes to RSI, slower is better. Touch-typing was designed for speed, not safety.

USE BOTH HANDS

In my opinion, the right-hand bias of the keyboard increases the risk of RSI for right-handed people, because certain common functions are designed to be performed exclusively by the right hand. To get around this, you can train yourself to use your left hand for some commands, and depressing the space bar. (People almost invariably favor one thumb or the other for spacing.)

It is awkward to reach across your torso for the number pad, for instance. My split keyboard has a detachable number pad, which also has Enter, Page Up and Page Down, and several other frequently used keys on it. Placing the number pad on the left side

The Origins of Touch-Typing

The beauty of touch-typing reveals itself in motion: Fingers know the placement of each key, the head balances lightly atop the spine, and arms move freely from the back and shoulders. Two-fingered typists must look at the keys, their heads bobbing up to screen, over to copy, and down to keyboard as they hunt and peck for keys, creating a literal pain in the neck.

Before I knew better, I marveled at the wisdom of this method. Surely the inventor of touch-typing had a brilliant sense of body mechanics, and prescience about the dangers of poor technique.

The premise that touch-typing was designed to protect the musculature, however tantalizing, is wrong. Mechanical expediency, not science, formed the basis for today's computer keyboard. Typewriter keys were arranged so that frequent letter pairs were separated to reduce the likelihood of jamming, thus allowing operators to type faster. Furthermore, typewriters were designed to be operated with the index and middle fingers because the other fingers were not considered very useful.

It was only a matter of time before someone challenged this notion, noted Darryl Rehr, editor of *ETCetera*, the magazine of the Early Typewriter Collectors Association in Los Angeles. One dissenter was Mrs. M. V. Longley, owner of the Shorthand and Typewriting Institute, who insisted that typists use all ten fingers instead of four. For this heresy, the press roundly attacked her. One article asserted that no one could type fast with ten fingers.

Frank E. McGurrin, another proponent of ten-fingered touch-typing, also disagreed. He considered himself the fastest typist around and challenged anyone to beat him at the keys. Louis Taub, a four-fingered typist who used the double keyboard, answered his dare. At the time, a battle raged over the shape of the keyboard: The Remington keyboard used the QWERTY layout with a shift key to make capital letters, whereas the Caligraph keyboard had two banks of alphabets, one lowercase and one in capital letters. Shift keys would confuse people, it was thought.

To settle the matter, a typing contest between the rivals was held in Cincinnati in the summer of 1888. McGurrin used a Remington, and Taub used the Caligraph.

"When they held the contest, there was no contest: McGurrin *smoked* Taub," declared Rehr. McGurrin sped ahead, eyes glued to the page, while Taub's gaze jumped from copy to keys and back. Not only did the duel prove that ten-fingered typing was faster than four-fingered, thereby changing the course of the future; it also doomed the double keyboard.

Instead of redesigning the layout, the standard computer keyboard follows the basic format of the typewriter keyboard, with the addition of important function keys. The manufacturers placed the new keys along the periphery of the alphabet, where they either require the use of the weakest finger—the pinkie—or force the user to stretch his or her fingers to reach them.

enables me to use both hands to execute these commands. It also allows me to use the number pad with my left hand. This way, I can balance the load between my overworked dominant (right) hand and my happy-to-help left hand.

EXERT ONLY THE EFFORT YOU NEED

Some people tend to get tense before activity—and stay tense during and after it. This wastes energy, impairs movement, and can be injurious. It is not enough to achieve the right posture and movement if you use enough force to crack the keyboard. Overabundant force or tension, such as pounding the keyboard or gripping a pen, destroys the benefits of good technique, because tense muscles overwork and become fatigued.

Instead, move like a cat. Use only the energy you need.

People who pound keys—or those with keyboards having little cushioning—might benefit from placing corn pads on their keys to soften the action. Write the corresponding letters on top of them.

Of Mice and Trackballs

If you really want to save your hands, avoid mice, trackballs, touchpads, and styluses. Software designers—while intending to make their programs "easy" to use—have done the public no service by forcing it to overuse the dominant hand. For people who do mouse-intensive work on a daily basis, such as graphic designers, the mouse can present a serious problem. It is tragic that these people have no choice about the tool they must use, and instead risk becoming permanently disabled.

Much as I dislike the mouse, I, too, am forced to use one because I have mouse-driven software, and there are no keystrokes to execute certain commands. On those rare occasions when I use the mouse, my technique is excruciatingly careful. For double-clicking, I use the Enter key.

Whenever possible, use key commands instead of the mouse. Memorizing common commands is easy if you use them all the time. Or tape a cheat sheet of frequently used functions on the monitor.

A Therapist's Back-Saving Tip

Occupational therapist Linda Johnson offers this tip to people who do computer training: Avoid leaning over anyone's desk to use the mouse. Instead, attach a mouse pad to a clipboard, balance the board in your free arm, then work while maintaining good posture.

If you absolutely must use a mouse, here are some pointers:

• When you click, drag, and circle the mouse over and over again, proper technique, good posture, and frequent stretch breaks are critical.
• Keep the mouse at elbow level so you can relax your neck and shoulder muscles.
• Move the mouse from the elbow, keeping the shoulder joint relaxed.
• Hold the mouse gently.
• Relax your thumb and pinkie.
• Finally, keep your mouse clean. Sometimes people grip their mouse because grit has gummed up the roller. If yours sticks, dismantle and clean it so you can roll smoothly instead of straining your muscles.

KEY COMMANDS FOR MOUSE-FREE MANEUVERING

Given the dangers of the mouse and trackball, it is much better to substitute keystrokes for click commands. Keystroke combinations for nearly all functions are embedded in the menu bar as a standard feature in many software programs. Look for the code alongside the word in the menu bar; for instance, "Control Q" is the code for quit. To see the codes, press the Alt key, and the menu bar will be highlighted. Using the arrows, you can move to the desired command, highlight it, and execute it with the Enter button instead of clicking the mouse. Glenn Devitt, a Webmaster, noted that most computer professionals actually prefer using key commands because this reduces interruptions caused by moving the hand from keyboard to mouse. Keystrokes produce more accurate movement as well.

Maneuvering the World Wide Web is more difficult; certain functions absolutely require a mouse. Still, some key commands exist, and many of these shortcuts work in other applications.

Back: Alt key and left arrow or Backspace key
Exit window: Control F4
Leave application: Alt F4
Minimize and maximize windows: Alt space, N or M
Highlight text: Shift key and arrows
Show all programs that are running: Control Escape
Previous field: Shift Tab
Scrolling: Arrow keys or Page Up/Down

Handwriting Technique

While some RSIers find handwriting more comfortable than computing, others find both activities intensely painful. Many people have sustained severe injuries from handwriting.

Even in our technology-ridden society, it is still easier to avoid computers than writing. All RSIers should assess their handwriting. If it hurts to hold a pen or write, you need to modify your habits.

GETTING A NEW GRIP

For most people, changing pen grips and handwriting practice is much more difficult than relearning computer or mouse technique. We usually learn to write at the age of five or six, so that by adulthood this habit has become ingrained.

However, with practice, a lot of patience, and hefty doses of motivation, it is possible to learn to write less stressfully. For people who need to write quickly—as do psychiatrists, reporters, and students—sometimes changes must be made incrementally.

"We must find ways of holding modern pens that will enable us to write fast without pain. Our hands were not designed to hold a small stick and make very accurate marks at speed and under stress," wrote Rosemary Sassoon and Gunnlaugur S. E. Briem in their book, *Teach Yourself Better Handwriting*. They offer the following suggestions:

• **The work space.**   Look at the area you generally use for writing. Is the table high enough? Perhaps an inclined writing surface would help. To see if this is more comfortable, put a clipboard on a small stack of books. Try slanting it tent- or easel-style.

• **Paper placement.**   Place the paper on the side of the body of the writing arm—that is, on the right side if you are right-handed, and vice versa. Aligning the paper with your torso cramps the movement of the arm.

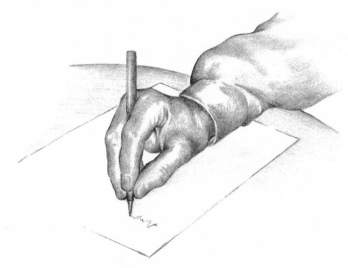

To use the alternative penhold, hold the pen between the index and middle fingers; this reduces the tension in the thumb and balances the use of tendons crossing the wrist and small muscles of the hand. Remember to hold the pen gently and stay relaxed as you write.

The Pen-Grip Test

Hunter Fry offers this simple experiment to show how much excess force it used in the act of writing: "Bring the tips of the thumb, index, and middle finger together in the most extended position. Now gently insert a pen, separating those fingertips (it is unlikely this is your normal pen grip). Keeping the fingers and thumb in that same position, holding the pen as lightly as possible, write two or three words slowly on a piece of paper. This will demonstrate how really little muscular effort is required to move the pen. Retain that memory and then compare your muscular effort after writing half a page in your normal way as fast as possible. The comparison between these two situations is so great that I once attempted to calculate the difference in muscle use. This rough calculation indicated that many writers would be using perhaps 100 times the muscle power that one actually needed to use."

• **Penhold.** Most people are taught a traditional penhold, with the pen held between thumb and index finger, balanced on the middle finger. This penhold works the muscles between the thumb and palm—and can be very painful if the pen is gripped tightly.

There is another penhold, where the pen is held between index and middle finger, with the thumb used as a guide. This instantly reduces the tension in the thumb and also releases tension in flexor tendons at the wrist. However, it requires some practice for everyday writing.

If you wish to learn an alternative penhold, practice when you are not under time pressure. Instead of trying to write words right away, make hatch marks and curlicues. Don't give up—it will be worth the effort if you can write more comfortably.

Voice-Activated Software

The vocal cords are subject to the hazards of overuse—speed, repetition, faulty posture, and poor technique—as surely as the hands. Lynda Marvin, a New York speech pathologist, noted that people who use voice-activated systems can experience chronic vocal fatigue and hoarseness.

Voice dictation systems can be balky, and users experience frustration not only from having to use them in the first place but also from commanding the system itself, according to John Haskell, another New York speech pathologist.

The chopped, discrete speech necessary to operate the system is itself considered vocal abuse. Additional risk factors for vocal problems include: lack of sleep, poor physical health, upper respiratory infections, colds, allergies, smoking, excessive alcohol consumption, shouting, and emotional or job-related stress. As with RSI, denial is also common with voice problems. Dr. Haskell said that people "have an episode, and get through it, and this cycle repeats itself until the voice gradually deteriorates."

If you are thinking of using a voice-activated program, first see a speech pathologist, who will show you how to correct speech patterns that over time may lead to distress.

SIGNS OF VOCAL DISTRESS

People who rely on their voices professionally can be vulnerable to vocal injury because of intensive use. Signals of problems include: strain, fatigue, weakness, effort upon talking, sounding hoarse or breathy, and pain.

We all have days when our voice may feel fatigued, but if there's a feeling of strain after an hour or two of talking, there's a problem. "Don't let it become chronic," Dr. Haskell advised. "Vocal problems can be serious. Get help immediately."

Tips for Vocal Athletes

- Take frequent breaks—at least every fifteen minutes or so.
- Keep your vocal cords moist by drinking lots of water. Drink water *before* you begin. Hydrating your vocal cords is not like watering your ferns; they get water from the bloodstream. Keep your throat moist by taking sips of water while dictating.
- Maintain relaxed, proper posture. A forward head posture or tight jaw puts tension on the muscles that suspend the larynx.
- Speak as smoothly as possible. Don't pound your voice. Instead, imagine you are speaking in connected phrases.
- Don't shout. Adjust the microphone so you can speak conversationally.
- Don't force a whisper. This can be as injurious as shouting. It could also be drying to the vocal cords, and the microphone may not pick up the voice, which adds to frustration and more repetition.
- Be aware of how you are using your voice in other situations. Eat in quiet restaurants and avoid noisy bars.
- Reduce the amount of talking you do.

Advice for Musicians

If God hadn't intended musicians to take breaks, He wouldn't have invented the intermission.

—ANONYMOUS

Playing a musical instrument presents many challenges. A wind or string player, in particular, must not only play the instrument but also support it while playing and lug it to the concert—a double whammy in terms of strain. Even the English horn can feel heavy, but imagine the tuba or cello!

PRACTICE SENSIBLY

"Music is ten percent hands and ninety percent brain. Don't practice too much," urged Dr. Markison, himself a working musician. That means no more than two hours a day of practice, interspersed with teaching, composing, arranging, performing, listening.

Tape practice sessions and listen to them critically rather than wearing out your hands.

TALK TO THE SOUND ENGINEER

When playing live, have the sound engineer boost the amplification rather than playing harder, and adjust your monitor so you can hear what you are playing.

RELAX AFTER THE SHOW

Performing can be stressful; even seasoned musicians get stage fright. Make sure you relax routinely. Sal Salvador, a guitarist who has played with jazz greats including Rosemary Clooney, Ella Fitzgerald, and Sonny Stitt, always unwinds by having dinner with a friend after the show. He swims and walks a lot, too.

He also makes sure he rests one day a week. "I forget all about this busy-ness," he said. "You must relax; otherwise you get uptight. If you get uptight, you have problems."

Tips for Safer Playing

PIANO AND ORGAN

- Adjust the height of the stool before you begin to play. (An organ bench cannot be adjusted easily. You may be able to raise your seated height with cushions or have a bench custom-made to your specifications.)
- Keep wrists neutral.
- Avoid ulnar deviation.
- Open the hand without stretching it for big chords.
- Allow gravity to bring the hand down instead of pounding the keys.
- The pinkie feels weak only when it is isolated. Use the power of the arm.
- Use fingering that is comfortable to your hand. Sheet music editors are not always the best judge of this.

DRUMS

Position your kit tightly around you, low enough so you do not have to lift your shoulders to play. A rack will help avoid many separate stands; it will also serve as a template so you don't have to redo positions from gig to gig. Adjust your stool so that you are sitting with your hips slightly higher than your knees and space your feet comfortably. Center yourself so you do not throw yourself off balance when you move your feet or arms.

If you are constantly splintering sticks, breaking drumheads, or cracking cymbals, you are playing too hard. If you think you are not getting enough volume out of the drum, get a new drum or increase amplification.

Notice how your hand responds to new instruments. "I changed to sticks that used a harder wood once," said drummer Glenn Devitt. "The new sticks were one-sixteenth of an inch smaller in diameter; everything else—weight, balance—was the same, but my hands hurt." Maybe Glenn had to grip tighter to hold the stick, or the different wood required harder playing. In any case, the pain went when the sticks did.

Joe Morello, a jazz drummer who has played with Marian McPartland, Stan Kenton, and Dave Brubeck, offered the following tips on how to avoid "stick shock":

- Don't keep the arms pinned to your side.
- Never hold the sticks to the head; rather, let them rebound like bouncing balls.
- Don't grip the sticks tightly.
- Play relaxed.

GUITAR

Jazz guitarist Sal Salvador, who has written over a dozen books on guitar technique, offered this advice:

- Don't play a guitar that is too heavy for you.
- If you use a strap, it should be padded and wide.
- Hold the guitar close to you, with your elbows relaxed by your side rather than winged.
- Make sure the strings are not too tight or too high off the fingerboard.

WIND INSTRUMENTS

- Musicians who have diminished or no sensation in their fingertips can glue a small round of fine sandpaper to the keys to increase sensation.
- Use a neck strap or mount so you do not have to support your instrument with your thumb.
- If your pinkie does not reach the stop of your flute comfortably, have an extension made.

———— 12 ————
CREATING YOUR NEW CAREER

Losing your job—especially if you have few financial resources to fall back on—can be terrifying. Job hunting, which most people find trying under the best circumstances, can be much harder when you have injured your hands. You may feel as if you'll never work again, much less find a job you love.

However, despite the difficulties, it is better to work than remain unemployed. Working is good for the psyche and good for the economy. Most people do not wish to stay home and withdraw from life; they want to contribute to society, not burden social services. The question becomes, how?

Deciding on a New Career

A friend said I got RSI because God had another plan for me. Couldn't He just have sent me a postcard?
—FRAN K., RSIer

As more and more people lost their jobs because of injuries, it became apparent that RSIers would be forced to take matters into their own hands if they wanted to work. It can be very discouraging to hunt for a job or change careers on your own, but what if RSIers joined forces with others who were also looking for work or thinking of starting their own businesses? They could be a valuable resource for each other; at the very least, they would understand what everyone else was going through. I decided to present a career workshop for RSIers to see what would happen. Sure enough, members offered valuable counsel to fellow RSIers, often pointing out hidden strengths or marketable talents to one another.

The Career Workshop

Any group of RSIers can use the methods in the Career Workshop. The workshop is roughly divided into three parts: some exercises to help you figure out what you want to do, a brainstorming session, and a plan to continue helping each other. Since job hunting is an ongoing process, make a sheet with everyone's name and phone number on it so people can contact each other when the workshop is over.

The workshop begins with a very important first step: believing you can find a fulfilling career despite your injury. Without this, it is impossible to do the work that follows.

Members are also charged with helping everyone else. They are encouraged to think of ways to help other RSIers fulfill their dreams, and discouraged from dissuading others from their goals. We get enough negative messages without adding any of our own.

THE PHILOSOPHY

Thinking of no-hands jobs sometimes forms the basis of jokes in RSI circles. For instance: You could be a rock star—assuming you have a miraculous voice, get promoted by Quincy Jones, and are not expected to play an instrument.

Levity aside, making a list is certainly one way to approach finding a new livelihood, but the focus of the Career Workshop uses another method: You figure out what you really want to do and then work at overcoming whatever obstacles stand in the way, rather than try to fit into an existing role.

STEP ONE: FANTASIZE ABOUT YOUR DREAM CAREER

People sometimes automatically assume their dreams cannot be fulfilled, so they refuse to think about jobs they would like. This is a mistake. Dream careers may seem impossible at first glance, but if you think about the obstacles long enough, solutions will often present themselves. Playing with ideas—simply fantasizing about how wonderful it would be to have your new career—encourages your subconscious to come up with a creative solution.

This attitude also opens up doors of opportunity, because instead of holding the thought "I can't," you have a positive outlook. People are far more likely to help you achieve your goals if you are not ambivalent about them yourself.

Actively fantasizing about an ideal career is the first step to achieving it.

STEP TWO: DEFLECT NEGATIVITY

Most people give up their dreams before they even take the first step to fulfilling them, usually because some significant person says they cannot have what they want. Do not let others project their own hopelessness and doubt on you. Believe in yourself no matter what anyone says.

Nine times out of ten, if people tell you what you want is impossible, it is because *they* do not think they could do something like that. This may be due to an emotional block of their own.

Sometimes people hold themselves back because they fear leaving other people in their life behind. A very wise woman once said, "You are the only person who can use your life." The fact that others choose not to pursue their own dreams or capitalize on their talents is very sad, but do not allow them to keep you from trying to reach important goals.

Unless they are insecure or jealous, other people usually want you to do well. They will generally be happy if you succeed, and someday they may tell you that you inspired them to try, too. So you can help others by setting a positive example by making yourself happy.

Listen to the people around you. Do they believe in you and encourage you to be fully yourself? Or do they put you down and disparage your ambitions? Choose friends who nurture you, help you grow, and want you to do well. Avoid people who hold you back.

STEP THREE: LOOK WITHIN

The following nine exercises are designed to elicit ideas for possible careers. Some of the questions are adapted from books such as *Wishcraft* by Barbara Sher with Annie Gottlieb, *What Color Is Your Parachute?* by Richard Nelson Bolles, and *Creative Visualization* by Shakti Gawain; others are my own. Put the questions on separate sheets of paper, and give yourself a few moments to answer them. If you cannot write, have someone help you, or answer the questions mentally.

One student of mine protested that the questions were far too profound to answer in the time allotted. I agree, and encourage you to take a lifetime if need be.

1. Make a list of your talents. List only the talents you enjoy using.

2. What do you value most in life?

3. Make a list of your best qualities. Be sure to include the comments of your friends. Don't be modest.

4. What is your proudest achievement? (This does not have to be career-related.)

5. If you were doing volunteer work, what would you do?

6. Based on the talents, values, and qualities you have listed in the previous exercises, describe your perfect day, from the moment you wake up until you go to bed. Include details: Where are you? What does your environment look like? What are you wearing?

The answer should be the height of your dreams. There are no limits to what you can do in your imagination. Money is no obstacle for the same reason. (Do *not* go on vacation. The beach gets pretty boring after a while, and this is a *career* workshop.)

7. State your life goal, then on the back of the paper write down any negative thoughts that come to mind.

For instance, write *"I could start my own business, but—"* On the back of the paper you might write: *"I don't have enough confidence." "I'm too lazy." "No one wants what I have to offer." "No one could start a company in this lousy economy." "Business is too competitive these days."*

The back side of the paper will help you uncover any internal blocks that prevent you from getting what you want. Once you are aware of them, they are easier to overcome.

8. How would you help someone else in your position achieve his or her goals?

9. If you could change the world, what would you do?

BRAINSTORM

At my Career Workshop, after everyone has had a chance to do the exercises, the floor is open to participants. One person describes her dream, then the group offers ideas or resources. If someone says she does not know what she wants to do, we look at questions one, two, and nine, where she describes her talents and what she enjoys doing and deeply values. Again, the group is asked to offer suggestions. This process continues until every member has had a chance to speak.

If you are brainstorming with a large group of your own, it is wise to divide the number of participants by the allotted time. For instance, if you have ten people and one hour of time remaining, each person would get six minutes.

Sometimes people have a lot of trouble finding a path. If you find yourself gravitating toward an activity, that may be a potential career direction.

One workshop student loved cats. "Why not be a professional cat-sitter?" another student suggested. Another attendee was intrigued with the saunterers of nineteenth-century Paris; she thought of giving tours of New York City's café society.

If, after some time, people still can't think of what to do with their lives, this generally falls into the category of mental blocks, because not knowing what you want to do is a surefire way of not being able to do it. If someone constantly says "I can't" or keeps coming up with excuses instead of moving forward with career plans, eventually the question becomes: Do you really want a job, or do you want to stay where you are?

The idea here is not to make excuses, but to find what you really want to do and build the courage to do it.

TAKE ACTION

Having a big dream is wonderful, but you need to take concrete actions to make it come true. Before people leave my workshop, everyone has to come up with at least one solid first step. This could be applying to school, calling a mentor, or joining a group that will bring you into contact with people who can help you. Anyone who is stuck may ask the attendees for suggestions.

REALITY CHECK

Sometimes a career can sound very appealing, but what happens if your dream doesn't match reality? For this reason, here is a final assignment for career-seekers. Talk to people in the field you want to enter, and find out what they actually do every day. For the price of lunch, you might save yourself years of study and educational costs. Or you might wind up bonding with someone who will act as your mentor.

STAY IN TOUCH

There are many good reasons to meet regularly with other RSIers to discuss your job search. You can be alert for job leads, resources, and information that another member of the group can use. You can partner with another RSIer to make sure you are each taking action in a job search instead of procrastinating.

When old-timers in the group report on what they have been doing to build their future, it can be very inspiring to newcomers. Old-timers can share their successes or seek additional ideas and support from the other members.

Talking About RSI on Job Interviews

Talking to a potential employer about your injury may seem like a surefire way not to get hired, but it can actually work in your favor. When Rekha Desai was looking for a new job, friends told her not to mention her injury. She decided to tell interviewers about it, because she didn't want the issue to come up later. "I had the atti-

Job-Hunting Hints

BUILD YOUR COURAGE

It takes guts to do what you want to do, especially when it means making career changes that involve a deeply personal dream that your closest friends may not realize you harbor. What if you fail? You might fear that you will be the laughingstock of your social circle. But would *you* laugh at anyone who tried to find happiness?

In fact, people admire those who do not sell out their dreams but instead make a genuine effort to realize them. Take a risk; even if you fail a few times, you will have the satisfaction of knowing you tried. Chances are, though, if you keep at it, you will succeed.

STAY MOTIVATED

It is hard to stay inspired when no one wants to hire you. Here, it is helpful to keep your heroes in the front of your mind. Read an inspirational book. Talk to a mentor. But don't give up. All it takes is one yes.

DO ONE HARD THING A DAY

When it comes to doing difficult things, many people tend to procrastinate. To avoid this tendency, do at least one hard thing a day. This was how Rome was built—brick by brick, one day at a time.

TAKE ADVANTAGE OF OPTIMISTIC MOMENTS

Just as we have good days and bad days with our pain, our emotions ebb and flow. As discouraged as you might feel, there will be days when you wake up feeling more energetic and optimistic than usual. *Take advan-*

tage of that feeling! Don't let it pass without making exploratory phone calls, sending out résumés, and taking positive action to get a job. Act when your positive energy is high.

THINK LIKE AN EMPLOYER

Put yourself in the manager's shoes. Would you want an applicant to call Monday morning after a holiday when you might be swamped, or late Friday when you're trying to get out of town for the weekend?

Sometimes the person in charge of hiring for a large company will be very pleased if you say, "You may not have an opening right now, but would you like to meet me in case one comes up suddenly?" Managers often hate hiring in a hurry, and this creates a less-pressured opportunity to evaluate you.

USE YOUR TIME WISELY

Do you spend your time as constructively as you can? Like money, time can slip away with little to show for it. While it is important to carve out some time for some soul searching, it is also important to spend time sending out résumés, making follow-up and exploratory phone calls, and doing such things as offering complementary samples of your services (if you are planning a business).

If evening comes and you realize you watched television for hours, dawdled over the paper, and schmoozed with friends all day, you need to concentrate on building self-discipline.

VOLUNTEER

There is nothing like being out in the world to take your mind off your own problems. Volunteering is a great way of getting experience doing what you think you want to do, and it beats sitting at home brooding. This experience may also tip the balance when you are trying to persuade employers to hire you, because it shows you are serious. You will also meet wonderful people this way.

tude that if the company didn't want to hire me knowing I have an injury, they were not a company I would like to work with," she said.

Rekha got three good offers and now works as a placement director for a company that specializes in computer-related jobs. "You would think companies wouldn't make job offers to injured people, but it was just the opposite," Rekha continued. "They appreciated the honesty. It impressed them."

Planning for Success

Several RSIers have successfully transformed their careers in ways that do not stress their hands. Dr. Piligian knows two people who embarked on careers that they had always wanted to do, and two others who did some of their best work after they were injured.

Gary Karp has given serious consideration to opening a flotation tank center. "It would be a place I'd make beautiful," he said. "I would create a sense of community." Providing a haven where people can reduce tension would surely make the world a better place, because, as Gary pointed out, "You can't think straight when you're tense."

Bob Hubbard has been playing music professionally for forty years. Most musicians in his position do many other things, he explained. When his injury became a problem, he took stock of the situation.

"Everybody except beginning students makes their own reeds. You can't buy good repair tools," he explained, so Bob learned to make them. "There are only two guys in the country who make tools that make reeds. I stepped in."

Now he plans to make tools for other reed players. He already does this at his home workbench. "If I had done nothing but play and had to put that down and do anything else, it would have been hard on me. Now it's just a question of doing less of one thing and more of another.

"I'm going to continue playing, but I may choose not to do certain kinds of work. I don't have to stop entirely. If I can't figure out how to make it work one way, I'll figure out another way," he said.

13

HESITATIONS ABOUT THE
INFORMATION SUPERHIGHWAY

When people say it is impossible to prevent repetitive strain injury, it reminds me of a comment someone made about the possibility of peace on Earth. "Just because it seems impossible doesn't mean we shouldn't *try*."

Computer technology is a fact of modern life. I would be a lot more enthusiastic about the technology if the tools people have to use were not so inherently harmful.

Most software requires initial learning time but becomes obsolete with each new version, which also needs to be mastered. This phenomenon is rather akin to learning a new language every six months. People spend an inordinate amount of time learning new programs rather than being able to focus on the job at hand. Many RSIers say their injury crested with the stress associated with a change of technology. New software also means you will be spending more time at the computer, another risk factor for RSI.

The Technological Treadmill

Every person who runs a business today is expected to have a modem, e-mail, and a Website—and whatever other new technology comes along. People who sank thousands of dollars into their current computer system groan that they need a new one because now their current hardware is not fast enough to support new software applications.

"I always remind people what the idea was around technology and computers in the sixties," said Gary Karp. "The first person to buy a computer was suddenly working faster than the competition, so the competition had to go out and buy a computer, too. Suddenly the turnaround time got shorter and shorter, and the expectations of how quickly things get done became the measure of whether somebody chooses to do business with you, and whether your business survives, or that the jobs exist. We weren't considering the impact on our lives and our health. We were thinking, 'Oh, great, we can go faster and faster.' "

SPEED IS STRESS

Technology imposes superhuman speed on all-too-human people. Across the United States and around the world, laborsaving technologies have revolutionized work. But instead of using our whole bodies at work, we depend more and more on our hands and arms. Computers have greatly contributed to this phenomenon, but technology has placed more work on the upper body in many other fields as well.

Prolonged high-speed work is quite dangerous to the body. It took millennia for our bodies to adapt to Earth's environment. We transgress the laws of Nature at our peril. By pushing ourselves beyond human limits, we risk irreparable damage to our hands. We need to reconsider the way we work, the tools we use, and think about the consequences of new technologies.

AMERICANS ARE OVERWORKED

A man who has a home office noted that e-mail and faxes do not invade your privacy the way the telephone does. After a late night, he sent a fax at 3:00 A.M. to a colleague who also works at home. He was astonished when he got back a response shortly after he sent the fax!

Twenty years ago—maybe even ten years ago—people took a lunch hour as a matter of course. They met friends, sat down at a table, and chatted while they ate. They did the same thing during coffee breaks. Nowadays, people grab sandwiches at their desk, working straight through the day.

Overwork pervades many occupations. Unless you are a professional musician, you probably would not think the staid world of classical music would be undergoing the same kinds of upheavals currently affecting corporations. But Bob Hubbard has noticed cataclysmic changes. "In the 1960s, even major orchestras played thirty-six weeks out of the year. Now all of the major orchestras and many second-tier orchestras work fifty-two weeks a year."

The Social Consequences of Technology

Advertisements for new technology almost invariably tout its ability to provide instant gratification. People become impatient with modems that require them to wait five minutes for e-mail—a feat that would have astonished our forebears, who relied on foot couriers and the Pony Express.

Is instant gratification always a good thing? On balance, maybe not.

For one thing, computers and other technologies are bad role models. If you do not dial a number fast enough, an irritating recording comes on and interrupts you. Or you dial a business number and you get lost in voice menus. Technology is literal and rigid. Humans can be intuitive and flexible. Computer programs do only what they are told to do. Humans are endlessly imaginative.

Human beings need human contact. One client of mine remarked, "You know, I have this vision that someday we're all going to be sitting alone in a room with hundreds of computers." His stark vision spoke eloquently of the loneliness inherent in working with computers. As messy, unpredictable, and difficult as human relationships can be, they are also the only way we can satisfy deep-seated needs for emotional connection to others.

While e-mail has been touted as a way of forming bonds with others, it seems highly artificial to some people. According to Susan Nobel, a social worker who runs an RSI support group at Mount Sinai Medical Center in New York, "People feel they have relationships with other people, but it's really a relationship with a screen. It's a screen, in more ways than one."

TOO MUCH RELIANCE ON COMPUTER USE
IS A DANGEROUS THING

People use computer technology now without even questioning whether it is necessary or good. I have polled respected doctors about how much computer use is safe for the average person. Two hours—with long breaks in between and proper technique, posture, and pacing—is a common reply. Most computer users spend three or four times that amount in front of the monitor.

Yet an escalating number of activities are computerized. People bank, buy stock, and book airline tickets online. Financial traders who used to watch for hand signals and write paper tickets now track a computer screen. Even the United Parcel Service driver has traded his paper log for a handheld computer.

Given the risk factors and increasing occupational and recreational computer use, the question is not *if* a lot more people will get RSI, but *when* they will get it. Granted, some young people can get away with long hours without seeming ill effect. But as they get older, prolonged computer use catches up with them.

Preventing RSI

Repetitive strain injury is a complex problem that requires a multifaceted response. No single entity can prevent RSI. There are several areas of responsibility, and they need to work together.

TOOL DESIGNERS

People who design tools should have a solid background in anatomy and kinesiology *before* they go to the drawing boards. At present, millions of people use tools designed by designers who appear to have little idea how the human body was meant to move. Any tool that requires prolonged use of the hand—from computers to hammers, drills, and dental and laboratory equipment—should be designed to protect the user. The same applies to household items from teapots to cleanser containers.

Once, after one of my lectures, a biology student showed me the instrument she used to perform delicate experiments. She had to squeeze a plunger repeatedly (and carefully, so she did not ruin her work) with her thumb. There was no way around the problem: she could not use both hands; nor could she always take a break for fear her experiment would be invalidated. And there was no other tool that would serve the same function.

This young college student already was experiencing warning

signs of RSI. She was risking crippling disability because of thoughtless tool design.

As consumers, we should speak up. Manufacturers know they must meet consumers' needs or they will lose business to competitors. They will design better tools when consumers demand them. Write letters. Call the consumer affairs department. Complain about dangerous design. Do not purchase shoddy tools when safe products are available to you.

PUBLIC AWARENESS AND EDUCATION

If people have never heard of RSI—much less know what the warning signs are—how can they prevent it? Tragically, instead of receiving treatment when injuries are reversible, many people don't respond to their symptoms until their injuries become permanent disabilities.

Children must be educated about the proper use of the hand and the upper body the very first moment they start to use computers in schools. Real physical education—in which children learn about anatomy, kinesiology, and the positive effects of exercise—should be taught in schools across the nation. While schools and politicians emphasize that children must be computer literate, it is even more important that children learn how to care for their bodies.

"Teaching is the most important job on earth," said Dr. Cianca. Whether by teacher or physician or coach, people have to learn proper posture and technique. "Even if the changes are subtle, it is better to always try to do things well than to give up and say it just doesn't seem to make any difference."

THE EMPLOYER'S ROLE

Employers can help prevent injury by providing adjustable workstations and chairs for their employees, and allowing self-pacing. Employees need to be able to stop *when they need to* rather than pushing beyond their physical capacity.

Employers should not be penalized for doing the right thing for their employees. It is distressing to hear about a company's plans to offer stress-management programs or ergonomics education being squelched because the legal department warns that doing so might be perceived as an admission of guilt if someone became injured. Companies willing to protect and promote employee health ought to be rewarded. It is heartening that many companies have put ergonomics plans in place.

THE EMPLOYEE'S ROLE

As more and more jobs combine sedentary behavior and repetitive motion, it is imperative that people maintain physical fitness to overcome the ill effects of their activities at work. Employees must take responsibility for keeping their body in good condition by consistently performing appropriate strengthening and stretching exercises. They need to maintain proper posture at the keyboard, use good technique, and take breaks routinely from repetitive work or static loading.

THE PHYSICIAN'S ROLE

Physicians can be a huge force for good in the effort to reduce the rate of injury by learning about repetitive strain injury. They can avoid prescribing drugs that might merely mask or suppress symptoms and help people recover in a thoughtful, thorough manner. Why prescribe an anti-inflammatory drug for a patient and then send that person back to the job without addressing the root of the problem? Doctors can intervene on patients' behalf, recommending good chairs and better workstations. Employers will sometimes provide equipment if it is recommended by a physician. They can help patients avoid reinjury by prescribing breaks, and by advising postural retraining and exercise. Doctors also have the power to put someone on temporary or permanent disability.

The Next Generation: Children and Computer Injuries

During the 1996 presidential campaign, Bill Clinton promised the nation to make sure every twelve-year-old could log on to the Internet. President Clinton is not alone in his enthusiasm for children using computers. You can hardly open a newspaper or watch television without someone extolling the virtues of making children "computer literate." According to a study by the Software Publishers Association, 62 percent of parents who have home computers and children under the age of six had purchased educational software for their youngsters. The children owned an average of six programs. Of the ten top-selling children's CD-ROMs, four suggest suitability for children beginning at age three. One program was designed for eighteen-month-old toddlers!

Many people appear to have embraced the notion that computers are good; therefore, the argument goes, children should be exposed to them early in order to be competitive and get good jobs. But the issue of children using computers raises serious concerns.

CHILDREN *ARE* AT RISK

Adults usually develop repetitive strain injury from a mix of poor posture, improper technique, faulty workstation setup, and inferior keyboard and mouse designs. If adults suffer computer injuries for these reasons, is it not logical to expect that children would also be at risk?

Some physicians suggest that children are protected from RSI because of growth hormones. But doctors and rehabilitation therapists tell me that they see younger and younger RSI patients. In any case, RSI results from cumulative trauma, so injuries do not occur overnight. Indeed, they may not appear until years later.

CHILDREN NEED PROPER WORKSTATIONS

Just as adults need proper workstations, so do kids. Small children are frequently pictured sitting in oversized chairs, arching their necks to look at monitors high above, and straining to reach the keys. A grossly inappropriate workstation can be very harmful to a child over time.

Don't Use Computers or Video Games in Lieu of Child Care

At one of my lectures on RSI, a woman asked me how to set up her two-year-old daughter's computer. To my knowledge, no one makes computer workstations for children that young. I asked the woman why her child had to use a computer.

Another mother supplied the explanation: "Why let her use the computer? To shut her up, because the child is *screaming* until Mommy lets her. She sees Mommy do it, and now *she* wants to!"

It is tempting to give in to a screaming child, but there are other activities for children that are much safer than computers.

Computer and video games present special problems. Anyone who has tried to pry a child away midplay knows how addictive these games can be. According to

GOOD POSTURE AND REGULAR EXERCISE ARE ESSENTIAL

Poor posture is extremely difficult to correct later in life. If children are not trained to stand and sit properly, to hold their spines erect— and if they are so out of shape that their muscles are not strong enough to do so—they are at a greater risk for computer injuries.

According to the 1996 *Surgeon General's Report on Physical Activity and Health:*

- Only about 50 percent of people between the ages of twelve and twenty-one regularly participate in vigorous physical activity. One-quarter of that age group do no vigorous physical activity at all.

an item in the *Orange County Register,* one fifth grader, Kristy Cameron of Newport Beach, California, refused to participate in a classroom assignment to give up television and video games for two weeks. "My life would be ruined without video games," she declared.

Children, like adults, become so engrossed in the action on the screen that they do not stop to take regular breaks. Why should they? They are having fun! The trouble is, they are forcing their hands through the equivalent of a marathon. When you combine awkward positioning, nonstop pounding, jamming, and gripping with poorly designed equipment, it is easy to understand how injuries can occur.

Handheld video games require the repetitive use of the thumb, which can lead to debilitating injuries years later. It is imperative to protect the thumb, because without it, the hand is virtually useless.

- As age increases, young people's participation in physical activity declines.
- Only 19 percent of American high school students engage in physical activity for twenty minutes or more in daily physical education classes.
- Among high school students, enrollment in physical education remained unchanged during the first half of the 1990s. However, daily attendance in physical education declined from approximately 42 percent to 25 percent.

PROPER TECHNIQUE MUST BE TAUGHT

Unless they are trained how to hold their hands, computer users rest their wrists on the table, which leads to a host of ailments. Children should learn proper technique from the moment they first

sit down at a computer. Good technique must be vigilantly reinforced until it becomes second nature.

CHILD SAFETY MUST COME FIRST

Nothing can stop the flow of modern technology, but parents and
teachers must not jeopardize children's future health in the rush to
provide them with a good time now or a job tomorrow. If we teach
children how to use computers they must be taught how to use
them safely.

---— *Epilogue* ---—

DISCOVERING THE GIFTS
OF RSI

Repetitive strain injury has many gifts to offer people who are willing to receive them. Once they overcome the anger and depression that often come with RSI, many people find inner peace and happiness they did not know before their injury. "Your values start to change," said Gary Karp. "Things that didn't matter to you before suddenly become precious."

Gaining Perspective

The great irony of our technological society is that no one has any time. As one of my friends put it: "All these people are rushing around, but where are they rushing to? Their death, ultimately!"

For many people, time out from the fray of the work world affords them the opportunity—perhaps for the first time since they were teenagers—to ponder life. They can contemplate their priorities and their values.

Any serious disease can put things in perspective. One student of mine realized that things that used to upset her did not bother her anymore. "I'm not so worried about losing five pounds or some stupid guy that didn't call me back," she said. "I'm not in such a rush to be successful," she added.

Another woman said she had learned she did not have to be perfect. Her goal was to live in the moment, to really listen when other people were talking, and to find peace within herself.

Others discover—or rediscover—the pleasures of a simple life. Our society, with all its laborsaving devices, allows us less and less time to just be. Louise M. saw the simplicity movement as a healthy sign and said that "people are getting off the treadmill. They realize they are addicted to consuming. I know a couple who spent money only on necessities and found it very liberating." One woman, who had been on the fast track in the computer industry, noted that before RSI, her life was a blur. Now she is thinking about the positive impact she can have on other people's lives.

PATIENCE

Patience is a hallmark of maturity. Instant gratification, on the other hand, reduces the human experience to the level of two-year-olds who throw tantrums when they cannot have what they want *right now*. People who do not embrace this valuable lesson sustain relapse after relapse until they do.

Lynette C. remarked that RSI was "a message from my body that for the last twenty-five years I have been driving myself at an inhuman level. I'm learning patience." Things like standing in line were not so onerous anymore. As Lynette explained: "My husband and I were on line in the grocery store, and he's usually very sweet, but he got impatient with the clerk because we had to wait. I thought, This is so silly."

TAKING TIME TO RELAX

Lynette C. discovered how to relax only after getting RSI. "I grew up with this incredible work ethic. My father worked morning, noon, and night. My mother worked. I have never had permission to relax before. RSI is the first time I've had to relax."

Because of her injury, Lynette also learned how to work in a more relaxed fashion. Instead of pushing too hard, she occasionally takes naps in the afternoon that leave her feeling refreshed and productive.

MODERATION

In our society, which values excess and overachievement, people are admired for working and playing too hard. Many people exercise with the idea of "no pain, no gain."

Overwork can take a toll on your personal life as surely as complete self-sacrifice to the family can breed resentment. We need to find the right balance of work, love, and play.

When Neill Rosenfeld first met his wife, he used to work twelve hours a day. "Now I want to be home. She can be working, I can be watching a video—it doesn't matter. I just want to be with her," he said.

Rediscovering the Joys of Human Relations

When was the last time a computer made you feel better when you were depressed? Computers cannot be kind to you. They cannot love you. They cannot sense your mood and say something soothing. Humans can. RSIers have a distinct advantage here, because rather than letting dehumanizing technologies tyrannize their lives, they can embrace more humane values and meaningful work.

As troublesome and uncomfortable as social interchanges can be, they are the only way to develop yourself as a person. "I feel like I'm gravitating more and more to people instead of technology," said Louise M.

Discovering Who You Are and What You Want

When she started out as a physical therapist, Sylvie Erb recalled, she was struck by how patients in their fifties and sixties with severe disease would tally their regrets about things they didn't do, or rue not seeing their kids grow up.

"Today many people go into a career track at the age of twenty—well, maybe fifteen now—and they never stop again to think of what they really want," said Sylvie. "There is only work—to be productive, to achieve more and more, to make more money. But it is not enough.

"It is better to discover who you are, and grow in that direction. It is important for people to ask, 'What *was* it I wanted to do with my life? Am I happy now?' People who find the answer have such a feeling of peace. They are grounded because they know what they want. Then the rest is easy."

Because RSI can affect people at a young age, it allows them more time to consider what sort of life they really want to live, she pointed out. Remember: You must take responsibility for your own happiness—no matter how dire the circumstances. This is a sign of wisdom and maturity.

VALUING HEALTH

During a conversation at a party, a man told me he had just had an important heart test performed. "I don't care if I live or die, I really don't. I just want to be healthy while I'm here," he said.

Would that more people felt that way—and took as good care of themselves as he did.

Repetitive strain injury often serves as a warning to people who have neglected their health. If they consequently modify their life-style, they can prevent many diseases that result from poor health habits. Take stock of your own health regimen. Are you as lean as you can be? Do you get enough appropriate exercise? Do you eat well? Sleep well? Are your relationships rewarding? Do you handle stress well? Little by little, you can replace negative health habits with positive ones.

LEARNING TO BE ASSERTIVE

One woman who had been very shy and afraid to ask for things she needed said RSI had helped her to become a more assertive person.

This can be as simple as requesting that tea be served in a smaller cup with easier-to-grasp handles. "I used to worry that the waiter might think I was neurotic or nutty, but now I don't care," said one RSIer.

BUILDING COURAGE

Louise M. said that she recently applied for a fellowship to study abroad for a year, something she never would have done were it not for RSI. Even going through the application process held a pleasant surprise; she got some "really nice references," she said.

FOCUSING ON THE QUALITY OF WORK

Speed does not necessarily bring satisfaction—especially when you enjoy the creative process. Louise M., a graphic designer, confessed that she missed the old days of tracing paper and drafting boards. "I got a lot of satisfaction out of doing a beautiful mechanical," she said. "I'm drawn to things that are finely wrought."

Quality work takes time, and people who return to simpler, slower tools such as charcoals, pencils, and paints will benefit not only by the fine patina of handwrought work, but will be able to ply their craft more safely because the tools are less dangerous. By working slowly, patiently, and with awareness of your body, you may find you can continue in your career or hobby without worsening your RSI. You can relish your work instead of rushing through it. Quality in one's work—and one's thinking—takes time, but working more slowly can often bring better results in the end because your projects will be well conceived instead of slipshod.

This could apply to many pursuits that are now computerized, such as graphic design, photography, and charting knitting patterns.

USING RSI AS A PATH FOR INNER GROWTH

Some people use physical ailments as a way to achieve emotional growth. For instance, if you were a very impatient person before RSI, you might be delighted to find that you are much more patient now. Maybe you were not as tolerant as you would have liked; having a disability of your own can increase your compassion for other people. Or perhaps you did not relate to others as well as you might have wished. Asking for help graciously can enhance your social exchanges.

RSI presents many opportunities to hone our inner selves. We can transform every obstacle into a challenge by asking: How can this work for me? We can triumph by applying our creativity to overcoming the problems we face. We can substitute new loves for old ones, instead of being consumed by regret and longing.

All in all, RSIers have a golden opportunity: Because we are not able to work at the same breakneck pace we once did, we have a chance to consider our lives. We have a perspective that is very hard to attain when you frantically chase one goal after the other.

One woman mused that our society is so achievement-oriented it is easy to feel left behind. But no one can duplicate anyone else's skills, sensitivities, talents. Only she can fulfill her destiny; therefore, in a very real sense, she has no competition. Each of us has our own unique gifts, though it is sometimes hard to remember this in a modular world where conformity is encouraged.

Qualities like wisdom, inner strength, patience, and compassion will sustain you through life storms better than any software program. I am counting on RSIers to help make this a better world—where work is more meaningful and humane and where human virtues are prized, and people create happiness by living up to their highest dreams.

Glossary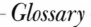

What Your Doctor Says and What It Means

Good doctors are willing to explain your diagnosis in plain English. As Dr. John Cianca puts it, "Patients aren't paying me to talk over their heads." Here are a few explanations of terms your doctor may have used that you might not understand.

Adson Test A test for thoracic outlet syndrome in which the pulse is taken at the wrist, while the patient's arm is lifted and his head turns.

Allen Test A test used to determine vascular impairment in which the doctor presses on both the radial and ulnar arteries, then lets go of one branch to test for obstruction in the other.

Anterior On the front of the body.

Apley's Scratch Test The patient is asked to try to touch the fingers of each hand between the shoulder blades as though pulling up a zipper, to test the range of motion in the shoulder joint.

Atrophy Wasting or withering of a muscle because it is not—or cannot—be used.

Bones of the Upper Extremity
Ulna, *radius, humerus, clavicle, scapula,* carpal and metacarpal bones, and phalanges.

Brachial Plexus   A network of nerves that originates in the neck and runs under the collarbone to control the hand, fingers, and arm.

Carpal Tunnel   A bracelet created by the *transverse carpal ligament* and carpal bones that encompasses the median nerve and nine tendons.

Carpal Tunnel Release
Surgery to relieve compression of the median nerve at the *carpal tunnel.*

Carpal Tunnel Syndrome
A compression of the median nerve at the *carpal tunnel* that can result in numbness and tingling of the hands.

Carpometacarpal (CMC) Joint or Basal Thumb Joint
The joint at the base of the thumb near the wrist.

Clavicle   The collarbone.

Cervical Radiculopathy
Injury to the nerves at their origins in the *cervical spine.*

Cervical Spine   The neck bones.

Cubital Tunnel Syndrome
An ulnar nerve entrapment that occurs at the elbow and can result from keeping the elbows bent or resting the forearm on a hard or sharp surface for extended periods of time.

De Quervain's Disease
An inflammation of the *tendon sheath* or *tenosynovitis* at the thumb near the wrist, often resulting from thumb intensive activities.

Deconditioned   Out of shape.

Degenerative Joint Disease (Osteoarthritis)
A common problem of the joints that can re-

sult from normal wear and tear, trauma, or overuse.

Distal Distant from the torso.

Dorsiflexion Bending the wrist so the top of the hand moves upward, as in the position of your hands if the wrists rest on the table during typing, or of a crossing guard halting traffic.

Double Crush Nerve compression along two areas on the same arm—for instance, both *cubital tunnel syndrome* and *Guyon's Canal syndrome*, or *thoracic outlet syndrome*.

Dupuytren's Contracture
A thickening of the fibrous tissue in the palm and fingers, which pulls the fingers toward the palm.

Electromyogram (EMG)
A test of the muscle's ability to respond to nerve impulses.

Epicondylitis An inflammation of the inner or outer elbow, commonly known to laypeople as tennis elbow, bowler's elbow, pitcher's elbow, or golfer's elbow, that can result from repeated *pronation* and *supination* of the forearms.

Extensor The muscles used to straighten (or extend) joints.

Fascia Connective tissue that surrounds muscles and other structures.

Fibromyalgia A chronic pain disorder that can include symptoms such as achiness all over, poor sleep, memory and concentration problems and fatigue.

Finkelstein's Sign A test for *De Quervain's disease*, in which you make a fist, and the doctor bends your wrist downward.

Flexor The muscles used to bend the joints.

Flexor Retinaculum or Transverse Carpal Ligament
A ligament near the base of the palm that holds the median nerve, tendons, connective tissue, arteries, and veins within the *carpal tunnel.*

Focal Dystonia or Writer's Cramp
A painless but debilitating condition in which the fingers make involuntary movements while performing certain tasks.

Frozen Shoulder   A term describing painful or difficult shoulder movement.

Ganglion Cysts   Small bumps that originate from wrist or finger joints or *tendon sheath,* frequently on the top of the wrist. Sometimes referred to as "Bible bumps."

Guyon's Canal Syndrome or Ulnar Tunnel Syndrome
Compression of the ulnar nerve at the wrist.

Humerus   The bone of the upper arm.

Hypermobility, Hyperlaxity, or Hyperligamentous
Overly flexible ligaments. The lay term for this is "double-jointed."

Iontophoresis   A modality used by hand therapists in which they apply creams containing cortisone solution to the skin, then rub an electrical device over the cream allowing the cortisone to penetrate through to the deeper tissues to reduce inflammation.

Lateral   Away from the midline of the body, as in outside the elbow.

Ligaments   Ligaments connect bone to bone.

Magnetic Resonance Imaging (MRI)
A diagnostic procedure in which a scanner takes pictures of the soft tissue to see if there is disruption to the structure, among other things.

Medial Close to the midline of the body, as in inside the elbow.

Muscles Muscles power and stabilize joint movement.

Myofascial Pain Pain of the muscles (myo) and connective tissue (*fascia*).

Neck Tension Syndrome
Irritation of the neck muscles, which can result from typing, carrying a load on one shoulder or hand, or holding the phone between ear and shoulder.

Nerve Compression, Entrapment, or Impingement
A condition in which the nerve is squeezed, usually by a muscle, tendon, or ligament.

Nerve Conduction Study
A test of the nerve's ability to conduct a signal.

Nerves Nerves conduct impulses from the brain to the body. Three major nerves of the upper extremity include the median, radial, and ulnar.

Neuropathy Damage to the nerve outside of the spinal cord.

Orthosis In the case of RSI, a splint or brace.

Phalen's Maneuver A test for *carpal tunnel syndrome*. Your doctor will ask you to press the backs of your hands together while bending your wrists for about a minute.

Phonophoresis A modality used by hand therapists in which creams containing cortisone solution are put on the skin. An ultrasound device is rubbed over the cream, allowing the cortisone to penetrate through to the tissue to reduce inflammation.

Posterior On the back of the body.

Pronation   Palms down, as in typing.

Pronator Syndrome   A condition that can result from median nerve compression stemming from strenuous flexion of the elbow and wrist.

Proximal   Close to the torso.

Radius   A forearm bone.

Range of Motion   The amount of movement possible in a joint.

Raynaud's Disease, Raynaud's Phenomenon, White Finger, Dead Finger, or Vibration Syndrome
                        A condition marked by cold hands because of spasm in blood vessels associated with gripping vibrating tools and/or working in a cold environment.

Referred Pain   Pain that originates from an area other than the part that hurts.

Reflex Sympathetic Dysfunction (RSD), Reflex Sympathetic Dystrophy, Sympathetic Mediated Pain Syndrome, Causalgia, or Complex Regional Pain Syndrome
                        A chronic pain disorder that may be associated with advanced RSI, surgery, splinting, or other conditions.

Repetitive Strain Injury (RSI), Repetitive Stress Injury, Repetitive Motion Injury, Cumulative Trauma Disorder, or Occupational Overuse Syndrome
                        Umbrella terms that refer to overuse injuries that occur to the upper extremity.

Rotator Cuff   A group of muscles—the supraspinatus, infraspinatus, teres minor, and subscapularis—that hold the *humerus* in place.

Rotator Cuff Tendinitis or Syndrome Supraspinatus Tendinitis, Subacromial Bursitis, Subdeltoid Bursitis, or Partial Tear of the Rotator Cuff
                        An inflammation, degeneration, irritation, or damage to the rotator cuff muscles or tendons.

Scapula   The shoulder blade.

Semmes-Weinstein Monofilament Test
A diagnostic test in which standardized nylon fibers are stroked on the palm and fingers to test the ability to feel light touch.

Sensory Impairment Loss of the ability to feel things normally.

Static Loading   Contracting muscles without movement at the joint, in a manner similar to isometric exercise.

Stenosing Tenosynovitis
A narrowing or constriction of the *tendon sheath*.

Subluxation   Looseness of a joint because of weakness in muscles or ligaments.

Sulcus Ulnaris Syndrome
An ulnar nerve disorder resulting from compression at the elbow.

Supination   Palms up, as in accepting coins.

Synovia or Synovial Fluid
A transparent lubricating fluid.

Tendinitis   The inflammation of the tendon, which is frequently associated with repeated motion and bending of a joint. In RSI, tendinitis can include bicipital tendinitis, rotator cuff tendinitis, flexor carpi radialis tendinitis, extensor tendinitis, and flexor tendinitis.

Tendon Sheath   A *synovial* covering of a *tendon* that allows it to glide through a tight area, as in the *carpal tunnel*.

Tendons   Tendons connect muscles to bones.

Tenosynovitis   An irritation that occurs when *tendon* and *tendon sheath* rub together. See *De Quervain's disease*.

Thoracic Outlet   The area between the collarbone, side of the neck, and shoulder that includes the *brachial plexus* and the arteries and veins that exit the neck to supply the arm.

Thoracic Outlet Syndrome, Anterior Scalene Syndrome, Brachial Plexus Neuritis, Costoclavicular Syndrome, Hyperabduction Syndrome, or Neurovascular Compression Syndrome

A compression of nerves or blood vessels of the *brachial plexus* in the *thoracic outlet* area. Symptoms include pain, numbness, and coldness of the fingers, hand, and forearm.

Tinel's Sign   A test for neurological impairment that involves tapping along a specific nerve.

Trigger Finger or Flexor Tenosynovitis

A condition in which a callous forms on the tendon and catches in the sheath, and the finger may lock in a bent position.

Trigger Points   Irritable areas within muscles that can cause local and *referred pain.*

Ulnar Deviation   The bent angle of the wrists as they reach sideways for the Shift, Enter, or Tab keys.

Upper Extremity   The hands, arms, and shoulders.

Vasculature   The arrangement of blood vessels of a body part.

Wright's Test   A test for *thoracic outlet syndrome.*

X Rays   Pictures of bones and used to diagnose arthritis, fractures, and bony abnormalities.

References

Page xi

"*The incidence of carpal tunnel syndrome . . .*", "Beating the Buzz of Carpal Tunnel Syndrome," Debra Page, *Pacific Fishing*, November, 1991, p. 117.

Page 2

"*The underlying premise for the term . . .*", "Upper Extremity CTD Management and Physical Assessment of the Upper Extremities," Ann E. Barr, Ph.D., P.T., Department of Physical Therapy, College of Allied Health Professions, Temple University, Philadelphia, Pa., and the Occupational and Industrial Orthopaedic Center, Hospital for Joint Diseases, a Member Organization of New York University Medical Center, New York, N.Y.

Page 4

According to the Bureau of Labor Statistics . . . , "Workplace Injuries and Illnesses in 1994," "Workplace Injuries and Illnesses in 1995," Bureau of Labor Statistics, U.S. Department of Labor.

Page 5

In 1981, there were 23,000 cases of RSI . . . , "Workplace Injuries and Illnesses in 1991," Bureau of Labor Statistics, U.S. Department of Labor.

Page 5

Consider the estimates . . . , "Cancer Facts & Figures—1995," American Cancer Society, Atlanta, Ga.

Page 5

According to . . . OSHA . . . , "Preventing Repetitive Stress Injuries," Occupational Safety and Health Administration, U.S. Department of Labor, December 10, 1996.

Page 5

As staggering as it is . . . , *Federal Register*, Vol. 57, No. 149, August 3, 1992.

Page 5

A University of California study . . . , "Reporting of Occupational Injury and Illness in the Semiconductor Manufacturing Industry," Stephen A. McCurdy, M.D., M.P.H; Marc B. Schenker, M.D., M.P.H; and Stephen J. Samuels, Ph.D., *American Journal of Public Health*, January, 1991, pp. 85–89.

Page 5

The estimated cost to business . . . , "Preventing Repetitive Stress Injuries," Occupational Safety and Health Administration, U.S. Department of Labor, December 10, 1996.

Page 5
According to a study of sign language interpreters . . ., "Biomechanical Factors Affecting Upper Extremity Cumulative Trauma Disorders in Sign Language Interpreters," Michael Feuerstein, Ph.D., and Terence E. Fitzgerald, Ph.D., *Journal of Occupational Medicine*, Volume 34, Number 3, March 1992, p. 258.

Page 6
The Stages of Injury . . ., "Upper Extremity CTD Management and Physical Assessment of the Upper Extremities," Ann E. Barr, Ph.D., P.T., Department of Physical Therapy, College of Allied Health Professions, Temple University, Philadelphia, Pa., and the Occupational and Industrial Orthopaedic Center, Hospital for Joint Diseases, a Member Organization of New York University Medical Center, New York, N.Y.

Page 11
"Of all the soft tissue injuries . . .", Soft Tissue Pain and Disability, Third Edition, Rene Cailliet, M.D., Philadelphia: F. A. Davis Company, 1996, p. 310.

Page 16
Spontaneous Healing: How to Discover and Enhance Your Body's Natural Ability to Maintain and Heal Itself, Andrew Weil, M.D., New York: Alfred A. Knopf, 1995, p. 61.

Page 16
"When a disease is uncommon . . .", "Personal Health: When Adrenal Gland Diseases Go Untreated, They Can Be Deadly," Jane Brody, *New York Times*, April 9, 1997, p. C10.

Page 24
"To many men, the need to visit . . .", A Man's Guide to Coping with Disability, Resources for Rehabilitation, Lexington, Mass., 1997, p. 12.

Page 25
According to the Surgeon General's Report . . . , "Physical Activity and Health: A Report of the Surgeon General," U.S. Department of Health and Human Services, Centers for Disease Control and Prevention, National Center for Chronic Disease Prevention and Health Promotion, the President's Council on Physical Fitness and Sports, July 1996.

Page 26
An average arm can weigh . . ., "Poor Posture Subjects a Worker's Body to Muscle Imbalance, Nerve Compression," Mary Lou Langford, P.T. *Occupational Health & Safety*, September 1994, pp. 38–42.

Page 27
The forward shoulder posture . . ., ibid.

Page 29
While sitting is the most frequent body posture . . ., Posture: Sitting, Standing, Chair Design & Exercise, Dennis Zacharkow, P.T., Springfield, Ill.: Charles C. Thomas Publisher, 1988, p. 51.

Page 29
Unfortunately, it is probably . . ., ibid., p. 51.

Page 32
In her study . . ., Stress, health, job satisfaction, Dr. Marianne Frankenhaeuser, Swedish Work Environment Fund, 1989.

Page 32
Another problem associated with high stress levels . . ., Musculoskeletal Disorders Among Data Entry Operators, by Robert DeMatteo, Margaret

Denton, and Lynda Hayward, WWDU '92, Berlin, 1992.

Page 32
In modern work, much physical stress . . . , Stress, health, job satisfaction, Dr. Marianne Frankenhaeuser, Swedish Work Environment Fund, 1989.

Page 33
Cigarette smoking increases your risk . . . , Circulation, Christodoulos Stefanadis, M.D., January 7, 1997.

Page 36
While phytochemicals have no nutritional value . . . , University of California at Berkeley Wellness Report: Nutrition 1994.

Page 36
Further, studies by the National Cancer Institute . . . , ibid.

Page 38
The Recommended Dietary Allowances . . . , Understanding Nutrition, Seventh edition, Eleanor Noss Whitney and Sharon Rady Rolfes, St. Paul: West Publishing Company, 1996, pp. 361, 363.

Page 38
According to the Tufts . . . , "For Carpal Tunnel Syndrome, Skip the B6," *Tufts University Diet & Nutrition Letter,* September, 1996, vol. 14, no. 7, pp. 1–2.

Page 47
Addiction to playing computer games . . . , "Stuck on the Web: The Symptoms of Internet Addiction," Pam Belluck, *New York Times,* December 1, 1996.

Page 49
"He jests at scars . . . ", William Shakespeare, *Romeo and Juliet,* Act II, Scene II.

Page 54
The amazing story of Jimmy Amadie . . . , "Jimmy Amadie: One Pianist's Triumph Over 35 Years of Disability," Robert Doerschuk, *Keyboard,* April 1994, pp. 96–97.

Page 61
Though overuse injuries were described . . . , "The Effect of Overuse on the Musician's Technique: A Comparative and Historical Review," Hunter J. H. Fry, *IJAM* 1(1), Fall 1991, pp. 46–55.

Page 62
"It seems extraordinary how little . . . ", ibid.

Page 65
Such drugs can have serious side effects . . . , Complete Drug Reference, 1993 Edition, United States Pharmacopoeia, Yonkers, N.Y.: Consumer Reports Books, 1992, p. 161.

Page 71
"Splints are used to immobilize . . . ", "Upper Extremity CTD Management and Physical Assessment of the Upper Extremities," Ann E. Barr, Ph.D., P.T., Department of Physical Therapy, College of Allied Health Professions, Temple University, Philadelphia, Pa., and the Occupational and Industrial Orthopaedic Center, Hospital for Joint Diseases, a Member Organization of New York University Medical Center, New York, N.Y.

Page 76
There are still a number . . . , Dr. Fulford's Touch of Life, Robert C. Fulford, D.O. with Gene Stone, New York: Pocket Books, 1996, p. viii.

Page 80
As Americans grow concerned about the side effects . . . , "Unconventional Medicine in the United States," *New England Journal of Medicine*, January 28, 1993.

Page 80
"When people who don't feel well . . .", "Something Old, Something New" *UCSF Magazine*, April 1997, p. 11.

Page 82
Biofeedback was developed in the late 1960s by . . . , "The Calm after the Storm," Deborah Quilter, *San Francisco Focus*, March 1984, pp. 57–101.

Page 87
This exercise is good . . . , Diaphragmatic breathing exercise, suggested by Prudence Ferraro, P.T., New York, N.Y.

Page 91
"[P]eople are already suffering . . .", Gerald W. Grumet, letter to the editor, *New York Times*, April 3, 1994.

Page 92
"I address myself to all the friends . . .", "A Petition to those Who Have the Superintendency of Education," Benjamin Franklin, from *Writings*, J. A. Leo Lemay, ed., New York: Library of America, 1987. (This essay also has been suggested as a parable for women's rights.)

Page 98
"At her favorite sushi restaurant . . .", Herb Caen's column, *San Francisco Chronicle*, May 4, 1994, p. D–1.

Page 98
Comedian Buddy Hackett explained . . . , *Shame and Pride: Affect,*

Sex and the Birth of the Self, Donald L. Nathanson, New York: W.W. Norton & Company, 1992, p. 392.

Page 100
"When I feel like exercising . . .", Robert M. Hutchins, *The Portable Curmudgeon Redux*, Jon Winokur, New York: Dutton, 1992, p. 101.

Page 101
"In a study of older people . . .", "Developing Optimal Exercise Regimes for Seniors: A Clinical Trial," Abby King, Ph.D., Stanford University Medical Center News Bureau Release, April 14, 1997.

Page 105
You are at risk of overtraining . . . , *Lifefit: An Effective Exercise Program for Optimal Health and a Longer Life*, Ralph S. Paffenbarger, Jr., M.D., Champaign, Ill.: Human Kinetics, 1996, pp. 316–317.

Page 105
Signs of overtraining include . . . , ibid. and *Strength Training for Women*, James A. Peterson et al. Champaign Ill.: Human Kinetics, 1996, p. 26.

Page 107
In his book . . . , *Spontaneous Healing: How to Discover and Enhance Your Body's Natural Ability to Maintain and Heal Itself,* Andrew Weil, M.D., New York: Alfred A. Knopf, 1995, p. 188.

Page 108
The human head weighs approximately . . . , *Soft Tissue Pain and Disability*, Third Edition, Rene Cailliet, M.D., Philadelphia: F. A. Davis Company, 1996, p. 215.

Page 110
If you must lean forward . . . , Posture: Sitting, Standing, Chair Design & Exercise, Dennis Zacharkow, P.T., Springfield, Ill.: Charles C. Thomas Publisher, 1988, pp. 363–4.

Page 116
Choosing the Right Tools . . . , "Occupational Overuse Syndrome: Checklists for the Evaluation of Work," published by Occupational Safety and Health, A Service of the Department of Labor, Wellington, New Zealand, first edition, August 1991, p. 18; "Human Factors in Occupational Medicine," Lawrence D. Budnick, M.D., M.P.H., *JOM,* Volume 35, Number 6, June 1993, p. 593; "The Ergonomics Manual: Guidebook for Managers, Supervisors and Ergonomic Team Members," Comprehensive Loss Management, Inc., 1990, p. 13.

Page 124
But before the invention of the printing press . . . , Memory Palace of Matteo Ricci, Jonathan Spence, New York: Penguin Books, 1985, pp. 2 and 9.

Page 125
New child-resistant caps . . . , "The State of The Art: Child-Resistant Packaging," *Pharmaceutical & Medical Packaging News,* February 1997, p. 58.

Page 126
This will also help some pharmacists . . . , Federal Register, Vol. 60, No. 140, July 21, 1995, p. 37727.

Page 130
Carrying Around Your "Bundle of Joy" . . . , "Preventing Wrist Pain When Caring for Your Baby," the Mount Sinai Sports Therapy Center, New York, N.Y.

Page 132
While cohosting a seminar on coping . . . , "How to Survive Your Computer: Staying Healthy at Work," conference sponsored by the New York Committee for Occupational Safety and Health (NYCOSH) and the Mount Sinai–Irving J. Selikoff Center for Occupational and Environmental Medicine, New York University, October 12, 1996.

Page 133
When men have limited . . . , A Man's Guide to Coping with Disability, Lexington, Mass.: Resources for Rehabilitation, 1997, p. 12.

Page 138
As . . . the authors . . . , Enabling Romance: A Guide to Love, Sex and Relationships for the Disabled (and People Who Care About Them), Ken Kroll and Erica Levy Klein, Bethesda, Md.: Woodbine House, 1995, p. 66.

Page 155
The Mouse Trap . . . , Some of this material originally appeared in "The Mouse Trap," Deborah Quilter, *VDT News,* July/August, 1995, p. 8.

Page 160
"While economists and Wall Street cheer . . . ", Annotation: Patients on the Auction Block, by Steffie Woolhandler and David U. Himmelstein, The Center for National Health Program Studies, the Cambridge Hospital/Harvard Medical School, *The American Journal of Public Health,* December 1996, Vol. 86, No. 12, p. 1700.

Page 164
"An eligible employee . . . ", Family

and Medical Leave Act of 1993, Section 2612, Leave Requirement.

Page 164

You may file a claim . . . , *Your Rights in the Workplace*, Barbara Kate Repa, Berkeley, Ca.: Nolo Press, 1994, pp. 14/6–14/13.

Page 175

"We must find ways of holding modern pens . . .", *Better Handwriting*, Rosemary Sassoon and Gunnlaugur S. E. Briem, Chicago: NTC Publishing Group, 1995, p. 42.

Page 176

"Bring the tips of the thumb . . .", "The Effect of Overuse on the Musician's Technique: A Comparative and Historical Review," Hunter J. H. Fry, *IJAM* 1(1), Fall 1991, pp. 46–55.

Page 186

The following nine exercises . . . , *Wishcraft: How to Get What You Really Want*, Barbara Sher, New York: Ballantine Books, 1979; *Creative Visualization*, Shakti Gawain, New York: Bantam, 1982; *What Color Is Your Parachute? A Practical Manual for Job-Hunters & Career-Changers*, Richard Nelson Bolles, Berkeley: Ten Speed Press, 1997.

Page 196

Financial traders who used to watch . . . , Face Lift at Board of Trade:

High Tech, Say Hello to Primal Instinct," Barnaby J. Feder, *New York Times*, February 17, 1997, p. 46.

Page 199

You can hardly open a newspaper . . . , Some of this material originally appeared in "Computer Injuries: The Next Generation," Deborah Quilter, *VDT News*, November/December, 1995, p. 8.

Page 199

According to a study by the Software Publishers Association . . . , "Software for Preschoolers Makes Market Inroads," by Andrew Trotter, *Education Week*, 1996, Vol. 16, Issue 15, p. 5.

Page 200

According to the 1996 Surgeon General's Report . . . , "Physical Activity and Health: A Report of the Surgeon General," U.S. Department of Health and Human Services, Centers for Disease Control and Prevention, National Center for Chronic Disease Prevention and Health Promotion, the President's Council on Physical Fitness and Sports, July 1996.

Page 200

According to an item . . . , "Fifth-Graders Find No TV a Tough Homework Task: She Just Won't Quit," Denice A. Rios, *The Orange County Register*, December 26, 1993, p. 16.

Other References

Pascarelli, Emil, M.D., and Deborah Quilter. *Repetitive Strain Injury: A Computer User's Guide*. New York: John Wiley & Sons, 1994.

Pećina, Marko M., Jelena Krmpotić-Nemanić, and Andrew C. Markiewitz. *Tunnel Syndromes*. Boca Raton: CRC Press, 1991.

Williamson, Miryam Ehrlich. *Fibromyalgia: A Comprehensive Approach*. New York: Walker and Company, 1996.

Resources

As with most consumer items, you get what you pay for. High-end products tend to be better constructed, easier to use—and costlier. If possible, try things out in the store before you take them home. You can learn a lot about a product this way. Beware of overblown ergonomic claims and shoddy merchandise. Look for money-back guarantees.

The following is only a sampling of resources available; you might find others on your own. The resources below are listed for your convenience and should not be considered endorsements. Prices were current at this writing.

Assistive Devices for Activities of Daily Living

CATALOGS

Ableware	(973) 628-7600
Access with Ease	(800) 531-9479
Access to Recreation	(800) 634-4351
Adaptability	(800) 243-9232
Ali-Med	(800) 225-2610
Enrichments	(800) 323-5547

TELEPHONE HEADSETS

Hello Direct	(800) 444-3556

READING AIDS

Levenger	(800) 311-4565

ADAPTIVE DEVICES

ABLEDATA
8455 Colesville Road
Silver Spring, MD 20910
(800) 227-0216

ABLEDATA is a database of thousands of assistive devices for activities of daily living. For more efficient service, tell the operator what equipment you need or which activities present problems for you rather than asking for general information about RSI.

Complementary Healing and Movement Techniques

ALEXANDER TECHNIQUE

North American Society of Teachers of the Alexander Technique
3010 Hennepin Avenue South, Suite 10
Minneapolis, MN 55408
(800) 473-0620

The North American Society of Teachers of the Alexander Technique (NASTAT) can provide you with the name of a teacher certified in the Alexander Technique in your area. NASTAT also has listings of Alexander Technique societies in foreign countries.

BIOFEEDBACK

The Biofeedback Certification Institute of America
10200 W. 44th Avenue, Suite 304
Wheat Ridge, CO 80033-2840
(303) 420-2902

The Biofeedback Certification Institute of America (BCIA) is a certifying body for biofeedback practitioners. BCIA will provide a list of biofeedback practitioners in your area.

The Association for Applied Psychophysiology and Biofeedback
10200 W. 44th Avenue, Suite 304
Wheat Ridge, CO 80033-2840

The Association for Applied Psychophysiology and Biofeedback (AAPB) is an interdisciplinary organization representing the fields of psychology, dentistry, nursing, physical and occupational therapy, and other disciplines. AAPB will provide the name of biofeedback practitioners near you if you send a self-addressed stamped envelope.

The Taubman Technique for Pianists
The Taubman Institute of Piano
Medusa, NY 12120
(800) 826-3720

Dorothy Taubman has developed a piano technique that has helped many piano students overcome arm and hand pain. The Taubman Learning Centers will provide the names of teachers trained in the Taubman Technique in selected cities. Videotapes of the Taubman technique are also available.

THERAPEUTIC TOUCH

Nurse Healers-Professional Associates Inc.
1211 Locust Street
Philadelphia, PA 19107
(215) 545-8079

The Nurse Healers-Professional Associates Inc. (NH-PA) will help you find practitioners and teachers of therapeutic touch in your area.

Government Agencies and Programs

U.S. Equal Employment Opportunity Commission
1801 L Street, N.W.
Washington, DC 20507

ADA Helpline (800) 669-EEOC (Voice) or
(800) 800-3302 (TDD)

The U.S. Equal Employment Opportunity Commission (EEOC) publishes free literature about using the Americans with Disabilities Act (ADA), and will provide the phone number of the office nearest you.

Job Accommodation Network
918 Chestnut Ridge Road
Suite 1
West Virginia University
P.O. Box 6080
Morgantown, WV 26506-6080
(800) 232-9675

The Job Accommodation Network (JAN) is a service that provides information and referrals about accommodating people with disabilities in the workplace. JAN advises on adaptive equipment and other accommodations and answers questions about the ADA.

President's Committee on Employment of People with Disabilities
1331 F Street, NW
Washington, DC 20004-1107
(202) 376-6200

Legal Assistance

Workplace Injury Litigation Group
P.O. Box 300488
Denver, CO 80203
(303) 830-0112

The Workplace Injury Litigation Group can provide you with the name of Workers' Compensation plaintiff attorneys in your area.

Nolo Press Self-Help Law Books and Software
950 Parker Street
Berkeley, CA 94710
(800) 992-6656

Nolo Press sells self-help legal books on everything from starting your own business, writing a will, consumer, and insurance issues, to solving workplace problems.

Newsletters

Repetitive Stress Injury Litigation Reporter
175 Strafford Avenue
Bldg. 4, Suite 140
Wayne, PA 19087
(800) 345-1101 (nationwide)
(610) 225-0510 (Pennsylvania)
Subscription price: $725 year; $435 six months
Covers legal issues related to RSI. Published monthly.

John Burton's Workers' Compensation Monitor
LRP Publications
747 Dresher Rd., Suite 500
Horsham, PA 19044
(215) 784-0860
Subscription price: $185 year

John Burton's Workers' Compensation Monitor is geared toward people who are interested in policy issues regarding Workers' Compensation. Published six times per year.

Nutritional Advice

The American Dietetic Association
National Center for Nutrition and Dietetics
216 West Jackson Boulevard, Suite 800
Chicago, IL 60606-6995
(312) 899-0040; (800) 366-1655 (Nutrition hotline)

The American Dietetic Association (ADA) can refer you to a registered dietitian near you.

On-line Information

Author's note: RSIers should carefully weigh the investment of hand energy expended in accessing on-line information against the potential benefits.

Sorehand

This is an archived, searchable forum for people interested in RSI. Subscribe by e-mail to: listserv@itssrv1.ucsf.edu. (and that's a one, not a letter el, in the domain name). The subject title may be left blank. In the body of the e-mail, write: SUBSCRIBE SOREHAND and your first and last name. For those who wish to keep their e-mail volume down, a daily digest is available: write SET SOREHAND DIGEST on the next line of the body.
To contact the list owner, use sorehand-request@itssrv1.ucsf.edu.

Deborah Quilter's WEB Site
http://www.users.interport.net/~webdeb/

This site contains basic information about RSI; back issues of the author's monthly *Computer Currents* column, "The Ergonomic Office"; a calendar of Deborah Quilter's speaking engagements and new developments in the field.

Osteopathy

Canadian College of Osteopathy
39 Altin Avenue
Toronto M4T2A7, Canada
(416) 323-1465

The Canadian College of Osteopathy has a trained number of practitioners who work in the United States and will provide you with the name of a practitioner near you. You may also travel to the school to be treated by a staff member there.

Physician Referrals

Association of Occupational and Environmental Clinics
1010 Vermont Avenue NW
Suite 513
Washington, DC 20005
(202) 347-4976

AOEC will refer you to an occupational and environmental clinic near you. The clinic may direct you to doctors knowledgeable about RSI or to support groups.

RSI Information

INFORMATION AND TECHNICAL ASSISTANCE

New York Committee for Occupational Safety and Health
(NYCOSH)
275 Seventh Avenue
New York, NY 10001-6708
(212) 627-3900

NYCOSH can provide you with fact sheets and technical assistance about coping with or preventing RSI, and Workers' Compensation issues. NYCOSH will also provide you with contact information for the Committee for Occupational Safety and Health nearest you.

RSI Support Groups

RSI support groups are often started at a grassroots level. Locations, times, and phone numbers can change, so information can become quickly outdated. However, Susan Nobel, who runs an RSI support group in New York City, is compiling a list of groups around the country. If you wish to receive information about a group near you, or would like your group added, contact her at:

Susan Nobel, M.S.W.
The Mount Sinai-Irving J. Selikoff Center
   for Occupational and Environmental Medicine
P.O. Box 1252
One Gustave L. Levy Place
New York, NY 10029-6574
(212) 241-1527
Enclose a self-addressed, stamped envelope.

You may also find a group through your doctor or physical therapist or by asking an uninjured friend to post a notice on an RSI bulletin board service such as Sorehand (see page 228). Or you can start one of your own and publicize it using the above networks.

Transportation

Ask your local public transportation system if you qualify for discount fares.

Sex Therapists and Counselors

American Association of Sex Educators, Counselors, and Therapists
P.O. Box 238
Mount Vernon, IA 52314-0238

Write for a list of licensed sex therapists and counselors in your area. Include a self-addressed, stamped envelope.

Sexual Aids Catalogs

Eve's Garden
119 W. 57th Street
Suite 1201
New York, NY 10019
(212) 757-8651
Catalog price: $3.00

The catalog may not list every device in stock, so ask if you have special needs.

Good Vibrations
938 Howard Street, Suite 101
San Francisco, CA 94103
(800) 289-8423

Xandria Collection: Special Edition for Disabled People
Lawrence Research Group, Inc.
P.O. Box 319005
San Francisco, CA 94131-9988
(800) 242-2823
Catalog price: $4.00

The Xandria catalog includes a great deal of educational material, especially the "Adaptations and Modifications" section.

Suicide Prevention

Suicide prevention hotlines are usually listed under community services, crisis intervention, or suicide prevention in the telephone book.

Further Reading

Drawing

Edwards, Betty. *Drawing on the Right Side of the Brain.* New York: Putnam, 1989.

Future of Technology

Stoll, Cifford. *Silicon Snake Oil: Second Thoughts on the Information Highway.* New York: Doubleday, 1995.

Handwriting

Sassoon, Rosemary, and Gunnlaugur, S. E. Briem. *Better Handwriting.* Chicago: NTC Publishing Group, 1995.

Healing

Weil, Andrew, M.D. *Spontaneous Healing: How to Discover and Enhance Your Body's Natural Ability to Maintain and Heal Itself.* New York: Alfred A. Knopf, 1995.

Job-Hunting and Career Changing

Bolles, Richard Nelson. *The 1998 What Color Is Your Parachute? A Practical Manual for Job-Hunters and Career-Changers.* Berkeley: Ten Speed Press, 1997. Revised and updated annually.

Bolles, Richard Nelson. *Job-Hunting Tips For the So-Called Handicapped or People Who Have Disabilities.* Berkeley: Ten Speed Press, 1991.

Hawken, Paul. *Growing a Business.* New York: Fireside, 1987.

Sher, Barbara with Annie Gottlieb. *Wishcraft: How to Get What You Really Want.* New York: Ballantine Books, 1979.

Optimism

Seligman, Martin E. P., Ph.D. *Learned Optimism: How to Change Your Mind and Your Life.* New York: Pocket Books, 1990.

Repetitive Sprain Injury

Pascarelli, Emil, M.D. and Deborah Quilter. *Repetitive Strain Injury: A Computer User's Guide.* New York: John Wiley & Sons, 1994.

Sexuality

Kroll, Ken, and Erica Levy Klein. *Enabling Romance: A Guide to Love, Sex and Relationships for the Disabled (and the People Who Care About Them).* Bethesda, Md.: Woodbine House, 1995.

Workers' Compensation and Workplace Rights

Ball, Christopher A. *How to Handle Your Workers' Compensation Claim: A Complete Guide for Employees.* Berkeley: Nolo Press, 1995. This book contains general information that would be useful to any claimant; however, it is specific to California law, so do not rely on the forms or certain instructions if you live in another state.

Repa, Barbara Kate. *Your Rights in the Workplace.* Berkeley: Nolo Press, 1994.

Index

Page numbers in italics indicate boxed text.

Acceptance, healing through, *88*
Acquaintances, 51
Action plan, 11–24
Acupuncture/acupressure, 80–82, 85
Addiction
  Internet, video, computer, 47, *200–201*
Aerobic exercise/conditioning, 34, 101
Airplanes, 130–31
Alcohol, x, 33
Alexander technique, 81, 83–84
Alignment, 102, 108
Alternative healing methods, 15, 80–81, 85
Ambidexterity, 90–91, *92–93*
Americans with Disabilities Act, 162–63
Anaphylaxis, 65–66
Anatomy, 31
Anesthesia, 69
Anger, 43
Antidepressant drugs, 43, 66–67
Anti-inflammatory drugs, 61, 65–66, 198
Antioxidant vitamins, 36
Antiseizure medications, 67
Anxiety, 9, 44
Applauding, *123*
Arm position, 26
Arthritis, 62
Aspirations, list of, *96–97*
Assertiveness, 206
Atrophy, 62, 71
Attitude, 10
Attorney(s), 162, 164

Automatic dialers, 128
Awareness, 10

Baby(ies), carrying, *130*
Back-saving tip, *173*
Bathroom remodeling, 126
Bicipital tendinitis, 4
Biofeedback, 38, 39, 81, 82–83, 85, 86
Blame, 49–50
Blood volume, 34
Body
  health regimens, 25
  keeping fit, 143
  tuning in to, 113
Body talk, 94–95
Body type, 31
Bone proportion, 31
Book trick, *111*
Bookmarks, weighted, 121
Books
  hardbound, 121
  on sexuality, 138
Boredom, 32–33
Brachial plexus, 26
Brainstorming (careers), 184, 187
Breaks, 158, 198
  frequent, regular, 17–18, 143–44
Breath trick, *87*
Breathing, x, 26, 29, 34–35, 145–46
  diaphragmatic, *87*, 89, 103
  shallow, *87*, 146

Briefcases, 127
Bulletin boards, 129

Carbohydrates, 36
Career(s), alternative/new, 159, 183–92
Career Workshop, 184–88
Carotenoids, 36
Carpal tunnel syndrome, 4, 5, 78
    laser treatments for, 75
    surgery in treatment of, 68–69
    vitamin B₆ in treatment of, *38*
Cars, 129–30
Cervical radiculopathy, 4
Chair(s), 27, 147–49, 197, 198
    choosing proper, *150*
    computer, *131*, 146
    reading, 121, 122
Childproof caps, 125–26
Children
    and computer injuries, 198–202
    education of, 197
    postural training, 26
Chinese iron balls, 90–91
Circulation, 29, 32, 33, 34, 99
Clothing, easy-to-wear, 127
Communication, in sex life, 136
Complacency, 19–20, 33
Complementary therapies, 81–85
    prescriptions for, 85
Computer equipment, placement of, 151
Computer games, 47, 144
Computer injuries
    children and, 198–202
Computer technique, 29, 77, 166–72
Computer technology, 193–96
Computer use, ix, x, 6, 7, 29, 30–31, 79
    avoiding, 113, 142
    downloading, 146
    overreliance on, 195–96
    shortcuts, 142
    sitting posture, 110
    upper-body strength in, 25
Computers
    as child care, *200–201*
    laptop, 155
Contrast baths, 70
Cooking tips, 118–19
Cortisone injections, 61, 67–68
Couch trick, *87, 89*
Courage, 206
Coworkers, 140, 157–58

Crowds, *23*
Crying, 53
Cubital tunnel syndrome, 4, 78
Cumulative trauma disorders, 2, 4
"Cures," 22–24

Dating, 133–35
Deep tissue massage, 70
Degenerative joint disease, 4
Denial, 8, 11, 42–43, 47
Depression, 43, 53, 57–58
De Quervain's disease, 4, 68
Desk accessories, 149–51
Devices, risky, 154–57
Diabetes, 35, 62
Diagnosis, 2, 10, 14
    and treatment, 12
Diary, *96*
Diet, x, 35–38, 116
Disability, xi, 9, 161, 164
    and discrimination, 162–63
    exercising with, 105
    and sexuality, 132–33
    telephone services for people with, 128
Disability insurance, 9
Do-it-yourselfer(s), 116
Doctor(s), 21, 86, 107
    avoiding wrong, 15–16
    role of, 198
    selecting good, 12–15
Doctor-patient relationship, 15
Doctor's visit, checklist for, *14*
Dominant hand, 90, 155, 156
    overuse of, 172
Dorsiflexion, 151, 166, 168
Dots, stick-on, 167–68
Driving, *23*
Drug containers, 126
Drug interactions, 65
Drug therapy, 65–68
Dupuytren's contracture, 4

E-mail, 194, 195
E. T. Handshake, *123*
Eating, 119
Education, x, 10, 70, 197
Elbows, 1, 64
Electroencephalogram (EEG) biofeedback,
    83
Emotion-washing technique, *56*
Emotional aspects of RSI, 41–60, 65

Emotional healing, steps to, 51–57
Emotional repercussions, 42–47
Employee, role of, 198
Employer(s), 140, 144, 158
  doctor's note to, 65
  role of, 197–98
  talking to, 157
Employment
  versus protecting hands, 158–60
Epicondylitis, 4, 68, 78, 141
Equestrian trick, *110*
Ergonomic equipment, 11, 21, 130–31,
  146, 147
Ergonomics/ergonomists, ix–x, 27, 197,
  198
Etiquette, *50*
Everyday life, specifics of, 116–24
Exercise, 10, 34, 61, 86, *96*, 198
  activities to avoid, 108
  cautions about, 105
  for children, 200–201
  daily workout, *106*
  with disability, 105
  in groups or pairs, 103
  healing power of, 99–111
  how to do, 102–3
  improper, *63*
  right amount of, 105
  RSI-friendly, 107
  solo, 103
Exercise program
  beginning, 100–105
  choosing, 101–2
  revising, 104–5
  sticking with, 103
Exercise triad, 101
Expressing emotions, 51–53
Extensor tendinitis, 4

Falling in love, *134–35*
Family and Medical Leave Act, 164
Fascia, 84–85
Fear, 44
  of losing one's job, 9
Fine motor coordination/skills, 26, 31
Fingers, 1, 65
  click, 155–56
  curved, 166–67
Flexibility, 31, 99
Flexibility training, 101
Flexor carpi radialis tendinitis, 4

Flexor tendinitis, 4
Flotation tanks, 89
Flower trick, *123*
Focal dystonia, 4
Folding papers, 129
Follow-up care, 65
Footrest, 149
Force, 30, 155
  overabundant, 172
Forearms, xi, 1, 64
Friends, x, 47, 48–49

Ganglion cyst, 68
Gender and response to RSI, 24
Gloves, 119
  fingerless, 87
Grieving losses of RSI, 46–47
Grocery shopping, 117–18
Growth, inner, 207–8
Guilt, 45–46
Guyon's canal syndrome, 4

Hand Bank, *115*
Hand dominance, 62, 90, 155, 156
Hand exercises/exercisers, 12, 108
Hand-grip/finger-pinch strength, 62
Hand-intensive activities, 108
Hand savers, *131*
Hand-saving, creative, *123*
Hand-saving principles, 112–16
Hand temperature, 62
  test for, 165
Hand use, ix, x, 5–7, 9
  monitoring, 79
  repetitive, 4
Hand-warming techniques, 86–87
Hands, xi, 4
  being kind to, 113
  cold, 31–32, 35, 68
  employment versus protecting, 158–60
  hypersensitive, 75–76
  misuse of, 165
  in neutral position, 166–67
  protecting, at work, 142–46
  protecting, during daily activities,
    112–31
  warm, 82, 90, 143, 165
Handwriting technique, 174–77
Head, weight of, 6
Head-forward position, 26, 27, 35, 63,
  108–9

Healing, 10, 25–40
 through acceptance, *88*
 deadlines for, 39
 elements of, 33–40
 emotional, 51–57
 exercise and posture in, 99–111
 natural, 34, 75
 patience in, 95–98
 readiness for, 85–86
Health, valuing, 206
Heart medications, 67
Height, 62
Help, asking for, 48, *52*
Herbal remedies, 22, 87–88
Heroes, *97*
HMO, 160, 162
Hole punches, 129
Home office, 128–29
Homeopathy, 80
Household tips, 124–26
Human relations, 205
Hypnosis, 82

Ice (treatment), 66
Imagery, 82
Information, unreliable, 20
Information superhighway, 193–202
Injury(ies), 4, 24, 25–40
 chain reaction, 76, 78
 chronic, 141
 compensatory/substitution, 78, 113
 elements of, 25–33
 hiding, 8–9, 11
 ignoring warning signs of, 33
 stages of, *6–7*
Injury-reinjury cycle, 20
Instant gratification, 195, 204
Insurance coverage, 74, 77, 84, 85
Interacting with other people, 47–51
Internet, 47, 142, 198–99
Interpreters, 5
Iontophoresis, 70
Ischemia, 27
Isolation, 47, 53–55

Job, quitting, 159–60
Job hunting, 183, 184
Job-hunting hints, *189–91*
Job interviews, 188–91
Job loss, 9, 183
Job-related injuries, 140

Job-related pain, 7–8
Jokes, *97*

Key commands (computer), 173–74
Keyboard, 22, 151–54, *170, 171*
 split, 151, 169–72
Keyboard support, 149–51
Keypad (telephone), 128

Laptop computer, 155
Lasers, low-energy (cold), 70
Laughter, 98
Lawsuits, 163
Learned helplessness, 32–33
Legal alternatives, 160–64
Leisure-time activities, 142–43
Lifestyle, x, 75, 206
Luggage, 131

Magnets, 22
Managed care, x, 74, 161
Massage, 11, 65, 81, 84, 85
Meals, preparing and eating, 116–17
Medical history and measurements, 62–63
Medical treatments, 12, 61–79
Meditation, 39, *56*
Memory aids, 124
Menopause, 24
Metabolites, 34
Microtrauma, xi, 7–8
Mirrors, 111
Mnemonic systems, 124
Mobility, stress and, 32
Moderation, 204–5
Motivation, 27, 98
Mouse (computer), 155–57, 166, 172–73
Mouse-free maneuvering
 key commands for, 173–74
Movement, 34, 108
 repetitive, 113
Movement reeducation techniques, 83
MRIs, 13
Muscle(s), x, 4, 31, 114
Muscle fiber composition, 31
Muscle strain injuries, 68
Muscle tension, 64, 91
Musical instruments, 179
 tips for safer playing, *180–81*
Musicians, 191
 advice for, 179–82

Myofascial pain, 4
Myofascial release, x, 84–85

Neck, xi, 1, 6, 26, 64, 107
Negativity, deflecting, 185
Nerve compression, 28*f*, 109, 146
    tests for, 64
Nerve compression syndromes, 68
Nerve entrapment disorder, 5
Nerve injuries, 4
Nerve testing, 64
Nerves, 29, 31, 35
Nonsteroidal anti-inflammatory drugs
    (NSAIDs), 65–66

Occupational overuse injuries, 3–4
Occupational physicians, 14
Occupational therapists, 86, 100
Occupational therapy, 65, 72–74
    types of, 70–75
Omega-3 fatty acids, 36
Opening doors, 114, 120
Opening packages, 129
Optimism, 56
Osteopathy, 76–77
Overtraining, 105
Overuse injuries, 61, 105
Overwork, *63*, 194–95, 205

Pacing, 10, 19, 39–40, 77, 140, 144–45,
    158
Page-turning devices, 121
Pain, 4, 9, 97–98, 141
    chronic, 8, 99
    in daily tasks, 8
    proper technique and, 165
    treatment of, 86
    as warning signal, 8, 17
    working in/through, 7–8, 17
Pain control/relief, x, 39, 74
Palpation, 64
Pampering, 89
Panty hose, 127
Paper placement, 175
Patience, 95–98, 204
Patient recovery checklist, *66–67*
Pectoralis (chest) muscles, 26
Pen expanders, 124
Pen grip, 174–77
Pen-grip test, *176*
Pencil sharpener, *131*

Penhold, 175*f*, 176–77
Personal care, 126–27
Personal plan (exercise), 101
Personal trainer, 103
Perspective, 203–5, 208
Pets, 89–90
Phonophoresis, 70
Physiatrists, 14
Physical condition(ing), 22, 31
Physical fitness, 198
Physical therapists, 61, 72–74, 86, 87, 103
    and exercise program, 100
Physical therapy, 12, 18, 65, 68, 77
    types of, 70–75
Phytochemicals, 36, 37
Pillows, 89, 119, 131
    reading, 121, 122
Positioning, awkward, 27, 155
Positioning hands, 30
Positive people, 55–56
Positive talk/self-talk, 57, 95
Positive thinking, 77, 81, 97
Postural retraining, 27, 63, 198
Posture, 63, 70, 140, 173
    in children, 26, 200–201
    healing power of good, 99–111
    practicing good, 111
    poor, 22, 26–27, 29, 34–35, 109, 177
    proper, x, 10, 108–11, 165–66, 198
    reading, 120–21
    static, 140
    therapeutic power of proper, 108–11
    while carrying things, 110
PPO, 160
Practitioner(s), choosing, 85
Pregnancy, 24
Pressure from others, 18–19
Prioritizing problems, 17–20
Productivity, 140, 158
Professional help, 51
    with exercise, 100–101
    sexual advice, 139
Programmable dialing, 154
Protein, 36
Psychological treatment, 13, 65
Psychotherapy/psychotherapist, 43, 51, 82
Public transportation, *23*
Purses, 127

Quality-of-life choices, 57–58

Radial tunnel syndrome, 4
Range of motion, 27, 62–63, 64, 65, 103
Raynaud's disease, 4, 66
Reading, 109, 120–21
Reading stands, 121
Recovery, x, 4, 10, 17, 22–24
    checklist, *66–67*
    length of treatment and, 74
    relaxation in, 91
    self-care in, 86
Recovery process, 25
    warnings about, 20–24
Rehabilitation
    returning to work after, 140–42
Rehabilitation therapy/therapists, 65, 70,
    80, 86, 105, 107, 108
    choosing, 71–72
    length of treatment, 73–74
Reinjury, xi, 141, 158
    preventing, 75, 143
    tendency toward, 78
Relapse, 19, 39, 45, 75–79, 142
    and exercise, 104
Relapse/healing/relapse cycle, 141
Relaxation, 91, 99, 179, 204
    deep, 94, 95
    self, 38–39
Relaxation techniques, *56*, 94
Relaxation tips, 95–98
Relaxation Workshop, 91–95
    homework for, *96–97*
Repetition, 22, 30, 155, 177
    voice, 152
Repetitive movements, 113, 140, 143, 198
Repetitive strain injury (RSI), ix, xi–xii,
    1–10
    as acid test, 135–36
    basics of, 2–4
    discovering gifts of, 203–8
    magnitude of, 4–5
    preventing, 196–98
Rest, 17, 34, *62*, 65, 75, 141
Right-hand bias (keyboard), 169
Risk factors, 21–22, 29, 42, 79, 144, 155,
    193
    vocal problems, 177
Rotator cuff tendinitis, 4
RSI; *see* Repetitive strain injury (RSI)
RSI examination, 62–65
"RSI personality," 41–42

RSI support groups, 53–55, 56, 65
    on-line, 20

Sanity, ways to save, 57–60
Saturated fat, 36–37
Scanners, 152
Scar tissue, 6
Second opinion, 70, 161
Sedentary behavior, 22, 25–26, 29, 198
Self-care, xii, 10, 70, 74, 86
Self-defense, *23*
Self-discovery, 205–8
Self-employed, 9, 143, 146
    problems of, 158
Self-help techniques, 86–90
Self-hypnosis, 82, 86
Self-medication, 8
Self-recrimination, 45
Self-relaxation techniques, 38–39
Self-splinting, 11
Self-treatment, 86
Serotonin, 67
Sex life, 132–39
    ten ways to better, 136–39
Sex therapist, 139
Sexual aids, 137
Sexual fantasies, 138
Sexual positions, 138
Sexuality
    as continuum, 136–37
    disability and, 132–33
Shaking hands, 122
Shame, 42, 45–46
Shoulder(s), xi, 1, 64
    frozen, 100
    high/low, 63, 110
    protracted, 63
Shoulder-forward position, 27
Side effects, 61, 65, 80
Significant others, 48–49
Silicone gel packs, 88
Sitting, 29, 99–100, 110, 145
Situations that require caution, *23*
Sleep, 38–39, 119
Smoking, x, 33
Soap dispensers, 126–27
Social Security Disability, 65, 164
Soft tissue injuries, 12, 13, 61
    reversal of, 141
Soft tissue manipulation/remodeling, 27,
    63

Software, 193
  see also Voice-activated software
Solo sex, 137–38
Soy products, 36
Special equipment, 65
Specialists, 14, 65
Speech, discrete, 152, 177
Speech pathologist, 177
Speed, 21, 30, 177, 207
  as stress, 194
Splints, 61, 68, 71, 119, 136
Sports medicine doctors, 14
Squeezing rubber balls, 61, 108
Standing position, 109
Staple removers, 129
Staplers, electric, 129, *131*
Static loading, 27, 29, 79, 100, 143, 152, 198
Strength test, 64, 65
Strength training, 101
Strengthening exercises, 77
Stress, 21–22, 32
  breaking cycle of, 91–94
  and cold hands, 31
  mental, 32–33
  speed as, 194
  symptoms respond to, 24
Stretching, 101, 173
Styluses, 156, 172
Success, planning for, 191–92
Suicidal thoughts, 43–44
Sulcus ulnaris tunnel syndrome, 4
Surgery, 61, 65, 68–70
Swelling, 63, 71
Swimming/pool aerobics, 107
Symptoms, 4, 8
  breaks and, 143, 144, 165
  emotional healing and, 60
  respond to stress, 24
Synovial fluid, 34, 99, 100, 102

Taking charge, 57
Tape recorder, 124
Tape Trick, *168*, 169*f*
Technique, 140, 152, 173, 198
  computer, 29, 77, 166–72
  faulty, 22
  handwriting, 174–77
  poor, 29–30, 155, 177
Technique, proper
  must be taught, 201–2
  at work, 165–82

Technological treadmill, 193–95
Technology(ies), 19–20, 21–22, 202, 205
  social consequences of, 195–96
Telephone, 127–28
Telephone dialing systems, 154
Telephone headsets, 65, 127–28, *131*, 147, 153–54
Tendinitis, 4, 5
Tendons, 4, 68
Tennis elbow (epicondylitis), 68, 141
Tenosynovitis, 4
Therapeutic massage, 84
Therapeutic touch, 81, 83
Therapies, new, 75
Thoracic outlet, 28*f*, 64
Thoracic outlet syndrome, 4, 35, 68, 78, 107
Thumb, xi, 65, 112, *201*
  sparing, *168*
Thyroid disease, 35, 62
Timing (exercise program), 102
Tobacco, 33
Tool designers, ix, 196–97
Tools, 10, 193
  choosing right, *116–17*
  hand-saving, 114
Toothbrushes, 127
Total-body workout, 102
Tote bags, 127
Touchpads, 156, 172
Touch-typing, 169
  origins of, *170–71*
Trackballs, 155, 156, 166, 172–73
Transcutaneous electrical nerve stimulation (TENS), 70
Trans-fatty acids, 37
Transverse carpal ligament, 69*f*
Trauma injuries, cumulative, 25
Travel, 129–31
Treatment, 10, 86
  comparing costs, 85
  complementary and self-care, 80–98
  diagnosis and, 12
  overview of, 61
  selecting, 85–86
  see also Medical treatments
Tricks and Tips for People with RSI (workshop), 112, 124
Trigger finger, 4
Trigger finger operations, 68
Trigger point injections, 67–68

TV watching, 121–22
Typing, 79
  hunt-and-peck, 168–69
  origins of touch-typing, *170–71*

Ulnar deviation, 151, 166, 167*f*, 168
Upper extremity, 1
Upper-extremity injuries, ix, xi, 4, 5

Vacation from RSI, 98
Victim, 57
Video addiction, 47
Video games, 143
  as child care, *200–201*
Vitamin B₆, 37, *38*
Vitamin C, 36
Vitamin E, 36, 66
Vitamin supplements, 22, 37
Vocal athletes, tips for, *178*
Vocal cords, 37, 152, 177
Vocal distress, signs of, 177
Voice-activated software, 30, 37, 152, 177
Voice dialing, 154
Voice systems, 151–54

Walking/hiking, 107
Walking trick, *145*
Warmth, 35
Warning signs, 1–2, 4, 39, 113
  ignoring, 33
Weight, 62
Wind instruments, *182*
Work
  giving up, 159–60
  interpersonal aspects of, 157–58

long hours, 30–31
proper technique at, 165–82
quality of, 207
returning to, after rehabilitation,
  140–42
therapeutic value of, 58
time off, x, 7, 17
Work ethic, 144, 157, 204
Work habits, 143–44
Work-related injury, 162
Work-related problems, 140–64
Work space, 175
Workers' Compensation, 9, 13, *14*, 51, 72,
  160–62
  claims for RSI, 5
  versus ADA, 163
Working in pain, 7–8, 17
Workload, reduced, 140, 141–42
Workout tips, *104*
Workstation(s), x, 10, 197, 198
  for children, 199, *200*
  proper, 146–47
  setting up, 148*f*
Workstation configurations/modification,
  22, 65, 140, 158
World Wide Web, 174
Wrist curls, 61, 108
Wrist position, neutral, 167*f*
Wrist-resting/rests, 22, 154, 201
Wrists, 1, 64
Writing, 122–24

X rays, 13, 64

Yoga, 39, 107